NUTRITION AND DIET RESEARCH PROGRESS

VITAMIN D: BIOCHEMISTRY, NUTRITION AND ROLES

NUTRITION AND DIET RESEARCH PROGRESS

Additional books in this series can be found on Nova's website at:

https://www.novapublishers.com/catalog/index.php?cPath=23_29&seriesp=Nutrition+and+Diet+Research+Progress

Additional E-books in this series can be found on Nova's website at:

https://www.novapublishers.com/catalog/index.php?cPath=23_29&seriespe=Nutrition+and+Diet+Research+Progress

NUTRITION AND DIET RESEARCH PROGRESS

VITAMIN D: BIOCHEMISTRY, NUTRITION AND ROLES

WILLIAM J. STACKHOUSE

Nova Science Publishers, Inc.
New York

For permission to use material from this book please contact us:
Telephone 631-231-7269; Fax 631-231-8175
Web Site: http://www.novapublishers.com

LIBRARY OF CONGRESS CATALOGING-IN-PUBLICATION DATA

Available upon Request
ISBN: 978-1-61668-273-6

Published by Nova Science Publishers, Inc. ✝ New York

CONTENTS

PREFACE

Vitamin D is a group of fat-soluble prohormones, the two major forms of which are vitamin D2 (or ergocalciferol) and vitamin D3 (or cholecalciferol). Vitamin D obtained from sun exposure, food, and supplements, is biologically inert and must undergo two hydroxylation reactions to be activated in the body. Calcitriol is the active form of vitamin D found in the body. Its major role is to increase the flow of calcium into the bloodstream, by promoting absorption of calcium and phosphorus from food in the intestines, and reabsorption of calcium in the kidneys. It is also necessary for bone growth and bone remodeling by osteoblasts and osteoclasts. This new book examines the biochemical components of vitamin D and the nutritional benefits it offers the human body.

Chapter 1 - Currently, there is increasing public awareness that vitamin D can do more than prevent rickets and otherwise improve bone health, but it still remains possible that some claims made in popular articles are poorly substantiated or exaggerated. Skepticism regarding vitamin D as a potential panacea is perhaps generated by the exceedingly high number of health benefits attributed to its ingestion or sunbathing, the anecdotal nature of the evidence in some cases, the lack of agreement on what constitutes the optimal levels of intake, and how exactly vitamin D produces better health. While there is considerable body of evidence suggesting that vitamin D may indeed have beneficial effects on a large spectrum of human disease, in part due to its immuno-regulatory properties, here we focus on the potential mechanisms that can explain how its optimal body levels can reduce the incidence of various human cancers, and on recent clinical studies of the effect of vitamin D and its derivatives on cancer cells. It is already well known that vitamin D can alter cell survival, in some cases inducing death of the malignant cells, and can reduce cell proliferation by blocking cell cycle progression. In addition, a variety of cancer cell types can be induced by vitamin D or derivatives to the more normal, non-proliferating, differentiated cells. This in some cases can be explained by the "Bypass-the-Lesion" hypothesis, according to which vitamin D allows an alternative lineage of cell differentiation of the malignant cells, the normal development of which was blocked by mutations that led to the emergence of the malignant clone, and then to a tumor. Thus, firm molecular grounds are emerging on which we can base our confidence that vitamin D, in an optimal daily dose of about 2,000 IU for most people, is an effective cancer preventive agent.

Chapter 2 - The structure of vitamin D was described by Adolf Windaus in 1927 (1). Brunette and co workers discovered that calcitriol is synthesized in the proximal convoluted tubule of the kidney (2). Slatopolsky et al suggested the role of active vitamin D in the treatment of secondary hyperparathyroidism (SHPT) (3). A lot of progress in our understanding of the physiology of vitamin D and its role in calcium and phosphorus homeostasis has been made in the recent years.

Chapter 3 - Vitamin D is a group of liposoluble components that organisms can obtain either via endogenous production from sun exposure or directly taken from foods and dietary supplements. In addition to its involvement in calcium metabolism, its presence plays other important functions in human health (e.g. reduction of inflammation and effects on cell proliferation and differentiation).

The discovery that most tissues and cells in the body have a vitamin D receptor and that several possess the enzymatic machinery to convert the primary circulating form of vitamin D (25-hydroxycholecalciferol, hydroxylated vitamin D3) to the active form (1,25-dihydroxycholecalciferol, calcitriol) has provided new insights into the function of this vitamin. Of great interest is the role it can play in decreasing the risk of many chronic illnesses, including common autoimmune diseases, cardiovascular disease, and cancers among others.

This chapter reviews the nature of vitamin D deficiency, its causes and effects on the human organism, and suggest strategies for its prevention and treatment by both natural sources and/or vitamin D supplements.

Chapter 4 - Vitamin D was identified as a curative treatment for rickets, a human disease causing bone abnormalities. Sunbathing was known to be effective for rickets treatment, and vitamin D was isolated as a factor activated by UV irradiation. Indeed, UV irradiation is required to convert the active form of Vitamin D, 1α, 25-dihydroxyvitamin D_3 ($1\alpha,25(OH)_2D_3$), from pro-vitamin D. Since 1α,$25(OH)_2D_3$ is required to maintain bone and mineral homeostasis, the ingestion of Pro-vitamin D from diet is also important for bone homeostasis. Shorter sunlight exposure or reduced pro-vitamin D intake causes rickets. Basically, 1 α,$25(OH)_2D_3$ is synthesized by metabolic conversions in the liver and kidney, and can bind to the vitamin D receptor (VDR) to express biological activities through modulating transcription of target genes. Functional deficiency of the 1 α,$25(OH)_2D_3$ metabolic enzyme and the VDR by gene mutations also results in vitamin D-dependent rickets. 1 α,$25(OH)_2D_3$ or its analogs have been used for treatment of renal bone disease and hyperparathyroidism, and later used for osteoporosis treatment as well. Osteoporosis, a disease demonstrating decreased bone mineral density (BMD) and loss of bone strength due to excessive bone resorption, has been treated with 1α,$25(OH)_2D_3$ and its cognate analogs. Treatment with active vitamin D_3 analogs is reportedly beneficial to correct abnormalities in mineral and bone metabolism in experimental animal models as well as in humans. Administration of active vitamin D analogs in ovariectomized (OVX) animals, a model for postmenopausal osteoporosis, reduces osteoclast number and bone resorption, thereby increasing BMD and bone strength. However, 1 α,$25(OH)_2D_3$ induces differentiation of osteoclasts, bone resorbing cells, in a co-culture of osteoclast precursor cells and osteoblastic cells *in vitro*. Treatment with 1α,$25(OH)_2D_3$ upregulates the expression of receptor activator of nuclear factor κ-B ligand (RANKL), an essential transmembrane ligand for osteoclastogenesis, while it downregulates osteoprotegerin (OPG), a decoy receptor of RANKL in osteoblasts, and that stimulates osteoclastogenesis in a coculture system. These discrepancies of *in vivo* and *in vitro* data make it difficult to understand the mechanisms underlying vitamin D_3 action on bone. Recent advances showed that 1α,$25(OH)_2D_3$ directly acts on the osteoclast precursor cells, and downregulates c-Fos protein, an essential transcription factor for osteoclast differentiation, or induces IFN-β, a strong inhibitor of osteoclast differentiation, thereby inhibiting osteoclast differentiation. These findings, at least in part, elucidate the anti-bone resorbing mechanisms of active vitamin D analogs in osteoporotic patients. In this context, the role of Vitamin D on bone metabolism including recent findings is discussed.

Chapter 5 - Vitamin D deficiency has been implicated in the pathogenesis of several disease processes ranging from autoimmune disease to malignancy. Knowledge in the area of vitamin D deficiency has grown exponentially over recent years, and relationships between vitamin D and many disease conditions, including benign and malignant thyroid disease, have been discovered. Thyroid tissue expresses vitamin D receptors and *in vitro* studies have shown that $1,25(OH)_2D$ (calcitriol) decreases proliferation and increases markers of differentiation in thyroid cancer cells. Vitamin D deficiency has also been found to have direct effects on thyroid function, playing a role in autoimmune hypo- and hyperthyroidism. This chapter will review the role of vitamin D in the thyroid by specifically looking at the function of vitamin D at the cellular level and its effects in both benign and malignant thyroid disease.

Chapter 6 - Magnesium (Mg) deficiency affects mineral metabolism in a dramatic fashion. Patients with severe Mg deficiency may present with increased neuromuscular hyperexcitablity characterized by paresthesias, muscle cramps and spasm, tetany, and seizures. This is thought to be secondary to profound hypocalcemia and Mg-deficiency induced decreased parathyroid hormone (PTH) secretion and PTH end-organ resistance, although low serum Mg concentrations can produce similar effects without concomitant hypocalcemia. More moderate degrees of Mg deficiency have also been linked to osteoporosis. Serum concentrations of 25(OH)-vitamin D have been observed to be low in patients with severe Mg deficiency and to be resistant to the administration of vitamin D metabolites. Similarly, serum concentrations of $1,25(OH)_2$-vitamin D are low in Mg deficiency. Experimental Mg depletion in humans and in animal models has resulted in a fall in serum $1,25(OH)_2$-vitamin D levels. This paper will review the evidence that Mg deficiency in both humans and in animals does adversely affect vitamin D metabolism and/or action

Chapter 7 - Topical creams containing vitamin D derivatives or analogues (calcitriol, calcipotriene) are currently used to treat different skin conditions including psoriasis and vitiligo with some success. The skin diseases that can be treated by topical vitamin D are characterised by irregular proliferation and differentiation of keratinocytes accompanied by inflammation and an influx of immune effector cells. We are now starting to better understand the mechanisms by which vitamin D applied to the skin affects keratinocyte growth and reduces the inflammation and immune responses, which drive these and other diseases. Here we outline some of the processes by which vitamin D modulates inflammatory processes that occur in diseased skin, and immune mechanisms that may be activated by vitamin D in the skin and draining lymphatic tissue to control inappropriate inflammatory responses. In particular, we focus on the cell-driven immune responses mediated by keratinocytes, dendritic cells and T cells that may be targets of vitamin D.

Chapter 8 - Oxidative stress is defined as an imbalance between the oxidant and antioxidant systems of the body. Olive oil is the main fat source in the Mediterranean diet which showed a protective role against ageing and/or oxidative stress and related diseases.

In order to investigate such *in vivo* effect on healthy human circulating cells, modifications of oxidative stress markers and platelet membrane fluidity before and after 3 weeks oral supplementation of 20 mL/day with Petrini Plus® were investigated. Petrini Plus® is an organic olive oil enriched with vitamins D3 (1,25-dihydroxy-cholecalciferol), K1 (phylloquinone) and B6 (pyridoxal 5 -phosphate).

15 healthy female volunteers (aged 25–40 years) were enrolled in the study. During phase 1 (3 weeks, T_1) subjects were provided with 20 ml/day of Petrini organic standard extra virgin olive oil, and during phase 2 (3 weeks, T_2) subjects were asked to introduce into their diet 20 ml/day of Petrini Plus extra virgin olive oil.

Thiobarbituric acid-reactive substances level (TBARS) decreased significantly in T_2 compared to both T_1 and T_0 as well as lipid hydroperoxide levels and conjugates dienes. Platelet membrane fluidity tested with probes TMA-DPH and DPH decreased significantly in T_2 compared to T_0 and T_1.

The results of present study suggest that the use, even though for a short period of time, of both Petrini organic standard extra virgin olive oil and Petrini Plus® oil in the diet of fertile women may have a protective effect against oxidative stress and provoke modifications in membrane fluidity of platelets. Moreover, the effects due to the supplementation of the enriched oil are more pronounced, thus confirming an antioxidant role played by the added vitamins (vitamins D_3, K_1 and B_6) and a preventing role against ageing and/or oxidative stress and theirs related diseases.

Chapter 9 - Vitamin D has become an intense topic of interest over the past 10 years. Vitamin D maintains normal blood levels of calcium and phosphorus and also aids in the absorption of calcium. Therefore, low vitamin D levels (25-OH vit D <30ng/mL) result in a reduction in intestinal calcium absorption, transient decreases in serum calcium, skeletal reabsorption, and a compensatory rise in parathyroid hormone (PTH). This is one form of secondary hyperparathyroidism. Recently, research also suggests vitamin D may provide protection from osteoporosis, hypertension (high blood pressure), cancer, and several autoimmune diseases [1, 2]. The recent interest in vitamin D stems, in part, from observations that inadequate levels of vitamin D are widely prevalent in society, with estimates of up to 36% in healthy adults and even higher percentages of elderly and hospitalized patients [3]. The high prevalence has been attributed to poor diet, minimal sunlight exposure, age-related decreases in cutaneous vitamin D synthesis and, possibly, the overuse of sun blocking products during outdoor activity [4, 5]. Hyperparathyroidism, which has a relatively increased prevalence in the aging population, can be complicated by co-existing vitamin D deficiency. We will explore the interrelationship between vitamin D deficiency and hyperparathyroidism in this chapter.

Chapter 10- Prostate cancer is a leading cause of morbidity and mortality among men in North America and northern Europe. [1]· Genetics, androgens, dietary and lifestyle factors have been recognized as contributors to risk of prostate cancer [2]· Epidemiological studies suggest associations between environmental factors and prostate cancer risk.

In: Vitamin D: Biochemistry, Nutrition ... ISBN: 978-1-61668-273-6
Editor: W. J. Stackhouse, pp. 1-35

Chapter 1

"VITAMIN D FIGHTS CANCER: FACT OR FICTION?"

George P. Studzinski[1] and Michael Danilenko[2]
[1]UMDNJ-New Jersey Medical School, Newark, NJ
[2]Ben Gurion University of the Negev, Beer Sheva, Israel

ABSTRACT

Currently, there is increasing public awareness that vitamin D can do more than prevent rickets and otherwise improve bone health, but it still remains possible that some claims made in popular articles are poorly substantiated or exaggerated. Skepticism regarding vitamin D as a potential panacea is perhaps generated by the exceedingly high number of health benefits attributed to its ingestion or sunbathing, the anecdotal nature of the evidence in some cases, the lack of agreement on what constitutes the optimal levels of intake, and how exactly vitamin D produces better health. While there is considerable body of evidence suggesting that vitamin D may indeed have beneficial effects on a large spectrum of human disease, in part due to its immuno-regulatory properties, here we focus on the potential mechanisms that can explain how its optimal body levels can reduce the incidence of various human cancers, and on recent clinical studies of the effect of vitamin D and its derivatives on cancer cells. It is already well known that vitamin D can alter cell survival, in some cases inducing death of the malignant cells, and can reduce cell proliferation by blocking cell cycle progression. In addition, a variety of cancer cell types can be induced by vitamin D or derivatives to the more normal, non-proliferating, differentiated cells. This in some cases can be explained by the "Bypass-the-Lesion" hypothesis, according to which vitamin D allows an alternative lineage of cell differentiation of the malignant cells, the normal development of which was blocked by mutations that led to the emergence of the malignant clone, and then to a tumor. Thus, firm molecular grounds are emerging on which we can base our confidence that vitamin D, in an optimal daily dose of about 2,000 IU for most people, is an effective cancer preventive agent.

INTRODUCTION

There is increasing general awareness that vitamin D can do more than just prevent rickets and otherwise improve bone health, but official recommendations for daily vitamin D intake still remain at the low levels of 400-600 international units (IU). This is contrary to the belief of many vitamin D researchers that in the absence of body exposure to abundant sunlight, although these levels may ensure skeletal health, they are insufficient to provide resistance to the development of neoplastic diseases [1,2].

While strong epidemiological evidence has been provided for this view, skepticism regarding its potential as an important component of regimens for cancer prevention persists. This skepticism is perhaps generated by the exceedingly high number of health benefits attributed to the ingestion of vitamin D and/or sunbathing, the anecdotal nature of the evidence in some cases, the lack of general agreement among scientists working on vitamin D what exactly constitutes the optimal levels of vitamin D intake, and precisely how vitamin D combats cancer.

Nonetheless, there is a considerable body of hard evidence suggesting that vitamin D may indeed have beneficial effects on resistance to cancer, as well as beneficial effects on a large spectrum of other human diseases. It is likely that the immuno-regulatory properties of vitamin D play an important role in its effects on all these diseases (reviewed in [3-5]), but here we focus on the potential cellular mechanisms that can explain how optimal body levels of vitamin D can reduce the incidence of various human cancers. In essence, evidence obtained using various human cell types indicates that the physiological form of vitamin D, 1,25-dihydroxyvitamin D_3 (1,25D), and its derivatives can eliminate or reduce tumor growth by promoting cell death by apoptosis, and/or retarding or blocking cell proliferation. Both cell cycle effects and apoptosis are in some case associated with the promotion of cell differentiation into more mature, senescent-like, phenotype.

1. EFFECTS OF 1,25D ON CELL SURVIVAL IN VARIOUS HUMAN CANCER CELLS

A very appealing mechanism for the elimination of tumors and hematological malignancies by 1,25D is induction of apoptosis, whereby 1,25D initiates programs that lead to cell death. Since apoptosis depends on the presence within the cells of a variety of cell death-executing proteins, such as the caspases, and the complex regulatory machinery upstream from the caspases, including members of the Bcl-2 family of proteins, death is usually selective for cell type. However, there are difficulties in a conclusive demonstration of apoptosis in many experimental situations, because the process is brief, requiring usually only a few hours, and the cell remnants (the apoptotic bodies) disappear, as they are phagocytosed and digested by adjacent cells and/or by professional phagocytes in the neighboring tissue. Nevertheless, a number of earlier reports presented evidence, based mainly on cultured cell lines, that 1,25D induces apoptosis in cells derived from human breast cancer [6-9], prostate cancer (eg, [10,11]), and colon cancer [12,13], but this may be dependent on low calcium levels in the diet when studied in animal models (eg, [14]).

A further potential problem in the translation of these in vitro results of the action of 1,25D on the enhancement of apoptosis is that most studies were conducted in vitro, using very high concentrations of 1,25D, usually 100 nM, which is more than three orders of magnitude greater than the serum levels of 1,25D. It is unclear if intracellular 1,25D concentrations at this level can ever be achieved. Also, it must be remembered that 1,25D has been shown to actually increase cell survival of several cell types, including keratinocytes [15-18], some bone-derived cells [19-22], and myeloid leukemia blasts [23,24]. In the latter, the increased cell survival in the presence of 1,25D may be related to the demonstrated increases in the activity of survival-enhancing kinases Erk1/2 [25,26] and Akt [27], and the recently described upstream regulator of MAPK cascades, the Kinase Suppressor of Ras-2 (KSR-2) [28,29].

Finally, there are difficulties in ascribing the epidemiologically observed anti-cancer effects of vitamin D to the induction of apoptosis, which was not uniformly observed in all cell lines derived from a given tissue, and the underlying mechanisms require more extensive studies. Nevertheless, even a small 1,25D-induced increase in the rate of spontaneously occurring apoptosis, especially during the early development of malignancy, could over the years contribute significantly to any anti-cancer effect definitively established for vitamin D, especially in susceptible organs such as breast, prostate and colon which, as it happens, are among the commonest sites of cancer in human populations.

2. Cell Cycle Effects of 1,25D on Malignant Cells

While the extent of 1,25D-induced apoptosis may be difficult to document as taking place in human tumors such as breast and prostate carcinomas, there is little doubt that the growth of these tumors can be inhibited or reduced by adequate concentrations of 1,25D. Indeed, this inhibition may result from a combination of apoptosis and reduced cell proliferation, as suggested by recent publications (eg, [30-32]). The hematological malignancy, acute myeloid leukemia (AML), provides a good model for studies of the mechanisms of cell cycle inhibition by 1,25D, which in this case is linked to monocytic differentiation of the malignant blasts [33]. An early observation using this system showed that the inhibitor of cyclin-dependent kinases (CDKs), known as p27Kip1, plays a major role in 1,25D-induced cell cycle block [34]. This finding has been replicated in many studies showing an association between up-regulation of p27Kip1 and cell cycle arrest in 1,25D-treated cancer cells (eg, [35-37]). The mechanism of 1,25D-induced p27Kip1 up-regulation appears to involve transcriptional activation of p27Kip1 gene expression via complex interaction between the nuclear vitamin D receptor (VDR) and the Sp-1 transcription factor on p27Kip1 promoter, which does not contain a canonical vitamin D response element (VDRE) [38,39]. Further insight was provided by the finding that p27Kip1 protein is stabilized by down-regulation of Skp2 ubiquitin ligase in head and neck squamous carcinoma cells [40], and was found to occur in other cell types, including ovarian cancer cells [41] and human hepatoma cells [42]. Of special interest, the expression of p27Kip1 in human AML cells can also be regulated at pre-translational level by microRNAs 181a and 181b, which are regulated by 1,25D in these cells [43].

In addition to p27Kip1, a related CDK inhibitor p21Cip1 is up-regulated by 1,25D in many cell types (eg, [35,44-47]), as well as somewhat less specific cell cycle regulators, such as the IGF binding protein-3 in prostate cancer cells [48,49], whereas telomerase is down-regulated in 1,25D-treated AML cells [50], the expression of which has recently been shown to be regulated as a multi-step process [51]. While most of the studies focused on the block in G1 to S phase transition, there are also reports of 1,25D-induced retardation of the G2 to M traverse, which can be associated with decreased levels of p34/cdc2 kinase [52,53]. Thus, there is abundant descriptive and mechanistic evidence that 1,25D can cause cell cycle arrest in a variety of human cancer cells.

3. Induction of Differentiation of Malignant Cells by 1,25D

Differentiation, whereby immature cells acquire the characteristics of functional cells of various lineages, can also account for anti-cancer effects of 1,25D on neoplastic cells. Induction of differentiation by 1,25D may take place in cells of prostate cancer (eg, [35,54-56]), breast cancer (eg, [57-60]), colon cancer (eg, [61-65]), and possibly some other solid tumors (eg, [37,66]). While the mechanisms underlying 1,25D-induced differentiation of these cells are known to a rather limited extent, in the past 25 years abundant evidence has accumulated showing many of the intricacies of how vitamin D and its derivatives signal monocytic differentiation of blasts from acute myeloid leukemia (AML).

The seminal observations originated in a series of publications from the laboratory of Abe and Miyaura in Japan showing that 1,25D and analogs induce differentiation of mouse and human myeloid leukemia [33,67], and this was further explored in laboratories in England (eg, [68-70]), Poland [71,72], and United States (eg, [73-77]).

Examples of those studies, taken from published work in the authors' laboratories, include the recognition that MAPK pathways participate in the signaling of 1,25D-induced differentiation, with ERK1/2 and JNK1/2 playing key roles (eg, [26,78]) , while p38 MAPKs alpha and beta having inhibitory roles [79]. Interestingly, there appear to be subtle interactions between the various MAPKs, as JNK2 appears to antagonize signaling of differentiation by JNK1, and this may account for the resistance of a strain of HL60 cells to

1,25D-induced differentiation [80]. Upstream, 1,25D appears to activate Raf-1, which is indispensable for this process [81,82], and the action of Raf-1, and perhaps also of other membrane-associated regulators, is modulated by the scaffold protein KSR-1, and its family member KSR-2 [28,29,83-85]. Downstream, the transcription factors identified as critical to 1,25D-induced differentiation of AML cells include AP-1 [86], C/EBPbeta [87-89], PU.1 [89] and MZF-1 [90]. These transcription factors then impinge on the regulators of differentiation and its functional proteins, such as CD14 and CD11b [90-92].

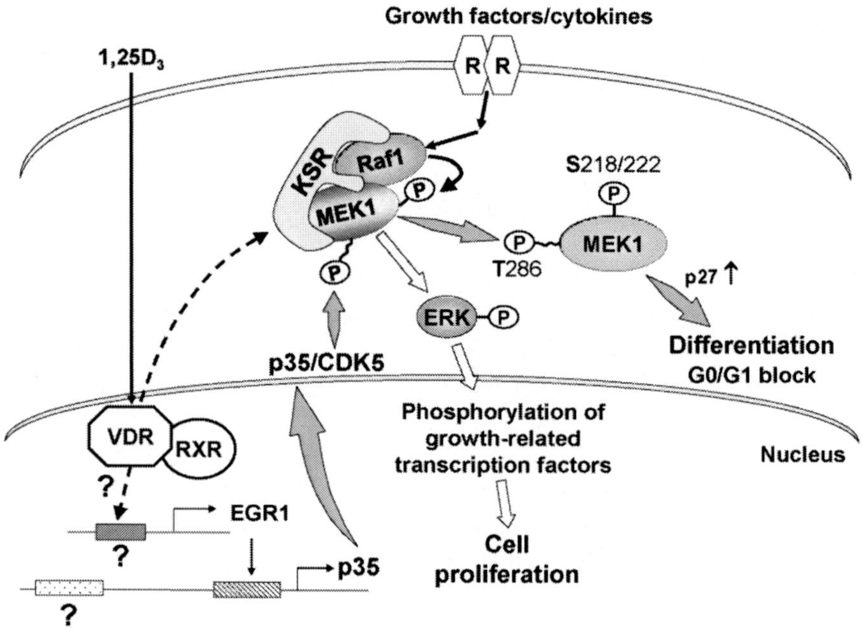

Figure 1. Schematic representation of the postulated role of p35 activator of CDK5 in the induction of differentiation-related block to the cell cycle traverse. VDR activated by 1,25D forms a dimer with RXR, which promotes expression of the transcrption factor EGR-1, and sequentially the expression of p35, a cyclin-like CDK5 activator. The p35/CDK5 complex can phosphorylate MEK1 on Thr286, which is an inactivating phosphorylation, and thus block transmission of the proliferative signal from Raf1. Also shown is the scaffold role of KSR-1, a direct VDR target, which participates in the MAPK cascade.

As mentioned above, differentiation is sometimes accompanied by apoptosis and always by cessation of cell proliferation, and when this is apparent it is referred to as "terminal differentiation". However, it is not widely recognized that in the case of myeloid cell differentiation the cell cycle effects follow, not precede, the morphological and functional differentiation [93], and can be experimentally uncoupled from the expression of differentiation markers [94]. A potentially important facet of the relationship between these processes is the finding that myeloid cells appear to be maximally sensitive to 1,25D at the interface of the G1 and the S phases [95]. A potential mechanism that links the 1,25D-induced changes in MAPK signaling may be an upregulation of the transcription factor EGR-1, which promotes expression of p35, an activator of CDK5 [96-98]. Since the p35/CDK5 complex phosphorylates MEK1 on T286 and thus inactivates it, this can explain the inhibition of cell proliferation by 1,25D and may involve p27Kip1 upregulation, as shown in Fig. 1.

4. THE "BYPASS-THE-LESION" HYPOTHESIS

Since the inability of cancer cells to achieve maturation, and thus to show evidence of differentiation, is generally attributed to structural changes in the cell DNA, *i.e.* mutations, which are irreversible, it seems remarkable that exposure of malignant cells to a vitamin can reverse the effect of mutations. We have proposed the hypothesis that the block to differentiation produced by a mutation of hematopoietic precursors can be by-passed by altering the balance of nuclear transcription factors in a manner that allows an alternate molecular route to differentiation [99]. Compounds such as 1,25D appear to act in this way. In the case of myeloid leukemia cells, the hematopoietic stem/progenitor precursors are unable to undergo granulocytic differentiation due to a variety of mutational events; however, the precursor cells retain the potential for monocytic differentiation, and since most of these express VDR, an exposure of such cells to 1,25D allows this form of differentiation. This may be achieved by increasing the level of C/EBPbeta [88], and perhaps other transcription factors, which allows the cells to bypass the block to granulocytic differentiation by becoming monocyte-like cells instead, as illustrated in Fig. 2. This scheme derives additional credibility from the finding that C/EBPbeta can interact directly with the promoter of CD14, one of the principal markers of monocytic differentiation [92]. Importantly, in freshly obtained AML-M2 leukemia cells exposed to a vitamin D analog, upregulation of C/EBPbeta paralleled the induction of monocytic differentiation [99]. Together, these data provide a basis for the hypothesis that deltanoid-induced upregulation of C/EBPbeta bypasses the block to granulocytic differentiation in the more primitive M2/3 myeloid leukemia cells by redirecting the cells to monocytic differentiation, or augments the action of 1,25D on differentiation-promoting transcription factors [100] in M4/5 AML cells which have minimal monocytic differentiation.

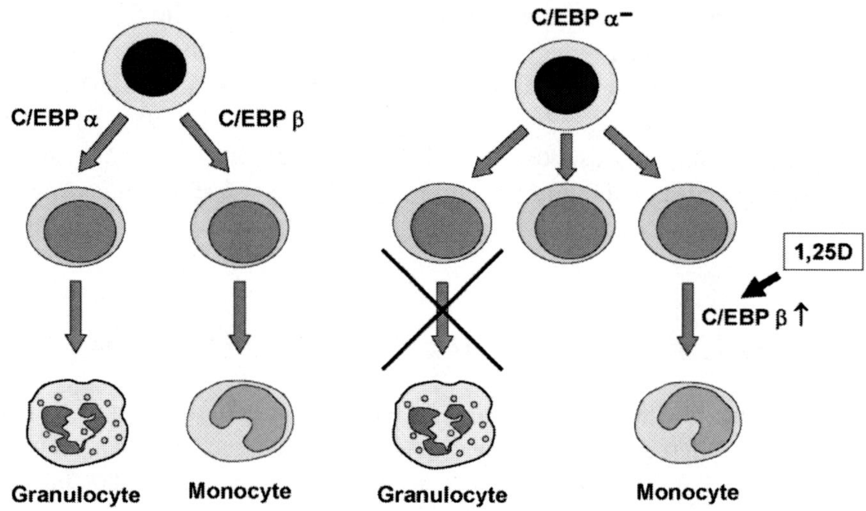

Figure 2. The "Bypass-the–Lesion" Hypothesis. Leukemia results from a block to normal hematopoietic differentiation in stem/precursor cells harboring mutations or epigenetic changes that block the expression of key molecules such as transcription factors necessary for differentiation. However, precursor cells often have potential for developing into more than one lineage of differentiation. In the case illustrated here, when granulocytic differentiation is blocked by lack of C/EBPalpha, an up-regulation of C/EBPbeta can redirect the mutated cells to monocytic differentiation, thus bypassing the block produced by the mutation. Experimental work has demonstrated that 1,25D can up-regulate C/EBPbeta, as discussed in the text.

5. Implications for Cancer Chemotherapy and Prevention

The demonstration of a marked antiproliferative and differentiation-inducing activity of 1,25D in various cancer cell types in both tissue culture (discussed in Sections 1-3 above) and animal models (eg, [37,101-105]) has suggested the potential therapeutic and chemopreventive significance of vitamin D compounds. This section provides an overview of the results of preclinical and clinical evaluation of 1,25D and its synthetic analogs in relation to different human malignancies.

a. Clinical Trials of 1,25D (Calcitriol)

Early trials in patients with myelodysplastic syndrome [106] and prostate cancer [107], in which 1,25D was administered daily at relatively low doses (1.5-2.0 μg), did not show clinical improvement. Hypercalcemia proved to be the major obstacle and limited the application of higher, pharmacologically active doses. Later, phase I/II trials in prostate cancer patients led to the development of a well-tolerated intermittent high-dose 1,25D regimen (45 μg weekly) [108] which, however, was not found to be effective as monotherapy (eg, [56]). On the other hand, encouraging results have recently been obtained with combinations of 1,25D and chemotherapeutic agents, such as dexamethasone [109], naproxen [110], docetaxel and estramustine [111] or dexamethasone and carboplatin [112], which demonstrated a significant decrease in prostate-specific antigen (PSA) blood levels in some patients. The ASCENT phase II trial of 1,25D and docetaxel also suggested an improvement in overall survival of patients with androgen-independent prostate cancer compared with docetaxel alone [113]. However, the following large phase III trial (ASCENT-2) has recently been terminated after enrollment of more than 900 men due to an unexpected increase in overall mortality in the 1,25D arm (reviewed in [114]). Thus, unconvincing results with 1,25D as the sole therapeutic agent support the necessity for combination therapy and the use of less calcemic vitamin D derivatives, as was outlined by Koeffler and colleagues as early as 1985 [106].

b. 1,25D Analogs

To date, thousands of vitamin D analogs (deltanoids) containing structural changes in the C,D-ring and/or the side chain region have been synthesized. A number of recently developed deltanoids have been shown to have significantly lower calcemic activity, as compared to 1,25D, while retaining the in vitro and in vivo anticancer properties of the parent compound (reviewed in [115,116]). Among these, MC 903 (calcipotriol) with a terminal cyclopropyl ring in the side chain [117], EB 1089 (seocalcitol) with a conjugated double-bond side chain structure [118,119], OCT (maxacalcitol), the 22-oxa-vitamin D_3 analog [120], and KH 1060, the 20-epi family analog [121] were found to exhibit growth- inhibitory and differentiation effects in a wide range of cancer cell types and to suppress the development of tumor xenografts in mouse models. Other examples of low-calcemic deltanoids with potent antiproliferative and differentiation-inducing activity include different Gemini analogs of 1,25D containing two side chains emanating at C-20 [122-126], 24-fluorinated hybrid analogs QW-1624F2-2 and JK-1624F2-2 [127-129], and 1α-hydroxyvitamin D_5, which contains an ethyl group at the C-24 position and lacks hydroxylation at the C-25 position [130,131] .

The therapeutic significance of several deltanoids has recently been evaluated in phase I/II clinical trials in patients with different types of cancer (reviewed in [116,132-135]). The major encouraging conclusion of these studies was that the analogs tested were indeed less calcemic than 1,25D in humans, and well tolerated at the pharmacologic doses comparable with those exhibiting some anticancer activity in preclinical studies. Although trials of EB 1089 in advanced cancer of the pancreas [136], breast and colon [137] did not demonstrate objective responses, a phase II study in patients with inoperable hepatocellular carcinoma has shown reduction in tumor dimensions, which was the first demonstration of the antitumor effect of a vitamin D analog in patients with an advanced solid tumor [138]. Clinical evaluation of the vitamin D_2 analogs paricalcitol and doxercalciferol in myelodysplastic syndrome [139,140] and androgen-independent prostate cancer [141-143] exhibited only limited activity of these compounds. However, treatment of benign prostatic hyperplasia with the fluorinated 1,25D analog BXL-628 (Elocalcitol) successfully arrested prostate growth [144]. Thus, despite limited overall progress in implementing deltanoid-based cancer therapy, some positive results warrant further clinical investigation of the antitumor activity of vitamin D analogs alone and in combination with other agents.

c. Combinations of 1,25D and Other Agents

Although, as described above, 1,25D and some of its less calcemic analogs have demonstrated both a marked antitumor activity in various experimental models and encouraging results in initial clinical testing, an ideal vitamin D compound that could be used as cancer medication has not yet been found. However, evidence accumulated over more than 25 years provides the basis for an alternative, combination strategy for vitamin D-based cancer therapy which may prove more effective compared with 1,25D or deltanoids administered as single agents. Initial observations made in 1983 by Japanese and Swedish research groups demonstrated a marked synergistic induction of differentiation in AML cell lines by near physiologic doses of 1,25D combined with the synthetic glucocorticoid dexamethasone [145] or the vitamin A derivative retinoic acid [146]. Since that time, numerous studies have confirmed the ability of 1,25D and its analogs to cooperate in the anticancer effects with various agents, in different experimental models of neoplasia (reviewed in [147-149]) and some clinical studies (discussed on p. 10). Here we present some recent successful examples of such cooperation.

(i) Differentiation-Inducing Agents

The fact that the nuclear vitamin D receptor (VDR) and the retinoid X receptor (RXR) interact to form a functional heterodimeric transcription factor (eg, [150]) suggests that vitamin D derivatives and retinoids, both being potent differentiation inducers, may cooperate in tumor suppression. Indeed, synergistic differentiation and antiproliferative effects of 1,25D combined with all-*trans* retinoic acid (ATRA) or 9-*cis* retinoic acid (9-cis-RA) have been reported in various cancer cell types (reviewed in [147,151]). Recently, 1,25D and 9-cis-RA have also been found to cooperatively inhibit lung carcinogenesis in the A/J mouse model [152]. Other natural differentiation inducers, such as protein kinase C (PKC) activators phorbol 12-myristate 13-acetate [153,154] and bryostatin-1 [155] synergized with vitamin D derivatives in the induction of AML cell differentiation and growth arrest.

(ii) Chemotherapeutic Drugs and Other Cytotoxic Agents

Since the discovery of their anticancer activity in experimental models, the idea of administering 1,25D and its analogs either as adjuvants or as integral part of conventional chemotherapy have attracted much interest. Indeed, a number of preclinical studies have shown that vitamin D derivatives potentiate cytotoxicity of chemotherapeutic agents, such as 1-β-D-arabinofuranosyl cytosine (Ara-C) in AML cells (eg, [156]) or cisplatin in a squamous cell carcinoma model [157]. 1,25D potentiated the effects of the antimitotic drug docetaxel in growth inhibition and apoptosis in androgen-independent prostate cancer cells [158]. Interestingly, combined treatment with docetaxel and 1,25D enhanced intratumoral immune responsiveness in animals bearing squamous cell carcinomas [159], thus demonstrating the potential of vitamin D derivatives for cancer immunotherapy. The analogs 24-ene-1,25-dihydroxyvitamin D_2 (PRI-1906) and (24R)-1,24-dihydroxyvitamin D_3 (PRI-

2191) cooperated with different cytotoxic and cytostatic agents, such as doxorubicin, cisplatin, imatinib and docetaxel in growth arrest of different cancer cell types [160,161]. Another deltanoid, paricalcitol, and arsenic trioxide were effective in the induction of differentiation and apoptosis of AML cells [162].

Recent findings demonstrate the enhanced induction of cancer cell death by the combined action of vitamin D derivatives and agents that induce oxidative stress. For instance, 1,25D sensitized colon cancer cells to H_2O_2-induced cytotoxicity [163], and menadione-induced depletion of the cellular antioxidant glutathione potentiated the apoptotic effect of 1,25D in breast cancer cells [164]. Interestingly, the deltanoid EB 1089 could selectively enhance breast tumor cell sensitivity to ionizing radiation [165], commonly known to act via generation of reactive oxygen species (ROS).

(iii) Epigenetically Active Agents

Several studies in hematopoietic, colon, breast and prostate cancer cells have indicated the ability of 1,25D to cooperate in the induction of differentiation and growth arrest with epigenetically active drugs, such as the demethylating agents 5-aza-2'-deoxycytidine [166] and decitabine [89] and the histone deacetylase (HDAC) inhibitors sodium butyrate and trichostatin A [167-169]. These data suggest that the transcriptional activity of VDR as well as certain key regulatory proteins involved in vitamin D signaling (eg, CDK inhibitors) are epigenetically suppressed in malignant cells [169,170], thus, providing the mechanistic basis for the epigenetic cancer therapy involving vitamin D derivatives.

(iii) Anti- And Pro-Inflammatory Agents

Vitamin D compounds have been shown to have anti-inflammatory activity (eg, [171,172]). Consistent with this, 1,25D cooperated with anti-inflammatory agents, e.g., non-steroidal anti-inflammatory drugs (NSAIDs), to enhance growth arrest in prostate cancer cells [173,174] and differentiation in AML cells [82,175]. In addition, 1,25D has been found to interrupt the production of the pro-inflammatory cytokine IL-1β in macrophages, thus inhibiting their ability to promote clonogenicity of colon cancer cells [176]. However, when administered together with the pro-inflammatory cytokine TNFα, 1,25D enhanced its cytotoxic effect in breast [177] and prostate [178] cancer cells.

(iv) Compounds that Inhibit Vitamin D Catabolism

25-Hydroxyvitamin D_3-24-hydroxylase (24-hydroxylase, CYP24) is a mitochondrial enzyme responsible for inactivation of both active vitamin D metabolites, 25-hydroxyvitamin D_3 and 1,25D. Therefore, CYP24 inhibition or downregulation would increase the half-life of bioactive vitamin D, thereby enhancing its cellular actions. Indeed, a broad-spectrum inhibitor of cytochrome P450 enzymes, ketoconazole, potentiated the differentiation and antiproliferative effects of 1,25D in AML cells [179] and cooperated with both 1,25D and its analog EB 1089 in growth arrest of prostate cancer cells [180]. Combined treatment of androgen-independent prostate cancer cells with 1,25D and the more potent CYP24 inhibitor, tetralone derivative-4, produced an enhanced growth inhibition [181]. Consistently, different agents that can downregulate CYP24 expression, e.g., 5α-dihydrotestosterone [182], HIV-1 protease inhibitor ritonavir [183] or ATRA [184,185], also potentiated the antiproliferative and differentiation activity of 1,25D in benign and malignant tumor cells.

(v) Phytochemicals and Other Natural Products

A number of phytochemicals have been reported to enhance 1,25D-induced differentiation in human AML cells (reviewed in [147]). Among these are the plant polyphenolic antioxidants curcumin, carnosic acid, and silibinin [186-190], sesquiterpene lactones parthenolide and costunolide [191,192], the natural triterpene betulinic acid [193] as well as the synthetic triterpenoid CDDO-imidazolide [194]. The ability to potentiate 1,25D-induced differentiation of AML cells was also demonstrated for several other natural agents, e.g., vitamin K_2 [195], the cardiotonic steroid bufalin [196] and the macrolide antibiotic nargenicin [197].

Different phytochemicals and other natural products have also been shown to cooperate with vitamin D compounds in non-leukemia, solid tumor cells. For instance, co-treatment with resveratrol, the phytoalexin found in red wine, enhanced the growth inhibitory effects of 1,25D and its analog EB1089 in breast cancer cells [198], while the soybean isoflavone genistein [199,200] as well as one of the most effective forms of vitamin E, RRR-α-vitamin E succinate [201], potentiated 1,25D-induced growth arrest in prostate cancer cells. In addition, fish oil enriched in ω-3 polyunsaturated fatty acids enhanced the antiproliferative effect of 1,25D on prostate [202] and liver [203] cancer cells.

The potential therapeutic significance of the combining vitamin D derivatives and other natural agents was supported by the findings that carnosic acid-rich rosemary extract and low calcemic 1,25D analogs 1,25-dihydroxy-16-ene-5,6-trans-cholecalciferol (Ro25-4020) and 19-nor Gemini synergized in the antileukemic activity in syngeneic mouse models of AML [204,205]. Furthermore, in prostate cancer xenograft models, RRR-α-vitamin E succinate enhanced the therapeutic efficacy of a tolerated dose of 1,25D without overt systemic toxicity or hypercalcemia [201].

The accumulated data indicate that the molecular mechanisms underlying the above cooperative effects involve modulation of various cellular systems. Thus, the phytochemicals carnosic acid, resveratrol and genistein [188,198,200], RRR-α-vitamin E succinate [201] and bufalin [196] have been shown to upregulate VDR expression and its transcriptional activity. Furthermore, genistein was found to directly inhibit CYP24 activity [200]. These two molecular events may explain the increased sensitivity of cancer cells to lower doses of 1,25D and its analogs observed in the above studies. Several studies, in AML cell lines have demonstrated a significant role of MAPK (eg, [129,154,187,190]) and PKC (eg, [187,192]) in the differentiation-enhancing effects of phytochemicals. Consistent with this, combined treatment with 1,25D and polyphenols resulted in upregulation and activation of MAPK- and redox-regulated transcription factors AP-1 [189,190] and EGR-1 [188,190], which are shown to be important for myeloid cell differentiation (discussed in Section 3). Since the VDR gene promoter contains two AP-1 binding sites [206], the VDR upregulation which occurs in this system may be due to 1,25D-stimulated AP-1 activity. This hypothesis is supported by the finding that treatment of AML cells with AP-1 decoy oligonucleotide resulted in a decrease in VDR protein content [86].

Collectively, the data generated in preclinical testing suggest that both 1,25D and at least some of its synthetic analogs can potentially be applied for cancer therapy. Phase I and II clinical trials conducted in patients with different malignancies have revealed safety limitations for these agents and provided the initial efficacy data, which allows continuing development of new treatment modalities. Accumulated evidence shows that a combinatorial treatment with vitamin D derivatives and chemotherapeutics or natural anti-cancer agents is a particularly promising approach which can provide a higher therapeutic efficacy compared with the compounds administered as single agents, and allows the use of lower, less toxic doses of these agents.

6. Conclusion

The evidence briefly, and of necessity somewhat selectively, summarized here, strongly indicates that vitamin D does indeed fight cancer. The clinical studies further support the conclusion previously based on the epidemiological studies and laboratory experiments that vitamin D is a major cancer preventative agent. Also, firm molecular grounds are emerging on which we can base our confidence that vitamin D, in an optimal dose of about 2,000 IU per day for most people, is an effective cancer preventative agent.

Acknowledgments

We thank Dr. David Goldberg, Professor Emeritus, University of Toronto, for his valuable comments on the manuscript. The authors' experimental work quoted here was supported by research grants RO1 CA 044722 and RO1 CA 117942 from the National Cancer Institute, USPHS.

Reviewed by Philip J Hughes, B Sc, Ph D.
School of Immunity and Infection,
College of Medical and Dental Sciences,
The University of Birmingham,
Birmingham, B15 2TT, UK.

References

[1] Studzinski GP, Moore DC. Sunlight--can it prevent as well as cause cancer? *Cancer Res,* 1995, 55: 4014-4022.

[2] Holick MF. Vitamin D and sunlight: strategies for cancer prevention and other health benefits. *Clin J Am Soc Nephrol,* 2008, 3: 1548-1554.

[3] Cantorna MT, Zhu Y, Froicu M, Wittke A. Vitamin D status, 1,25-dihydroxyvitamin D_3, and the immune system. *Am J Clin Nutr*, 2004, 80: 1717S-1720S.

[4] Baeke F, van Etten E, Gysemans C, Overbergh L, Mathieu C. Vitamin D signaling in immune-mediated disorders: Evolving insights and therapeutic opportunities. *Mol Aspects Med*, 2008, 29: 376-387.

[5] Adams JS, Hewison M. Unexpected actions of vitamin D: new perspectives on the regulation of innate and adaptive immunity. *Nat Clin Pract Endocrinol Metab*, 2008, 4: 80-90.

[6] James SY, Mackay AG, Colston KW. Vitamin D derivatives in combination with 9-cis retinoic acid promote active cell death in breast cancer cells. *J Mol Endocrinol,* 1995, 14: 391-394.

[7] Simboli-Campbell M, Narvaez CJ, Tenniswood M, Welsh J. 1,25-Dihydroxyvitamin D_3 induces morphological and biochemical markers of apoptosis in MCF-7 breast cancer cells. *J Steroid Biochem Mol Biol*, 1996, 58: 367-376.

[8] Hansen CM, Rohde L, Madsen MW, Hansen D, Colston KW, Pirianov G, Holm PK, Binderup L. MCF-7/VD(R): a new vitamin D resistant cell line. *J Cell Biochem,* 2001, 82: 422-436.

[9] Colston KW, Hansen CM. Mechanisms implicated in the growth regulatory effects of vitamin D in breast cancer. *Endocr Relat Cancer*, 2002, 9: 45-59.

[10] Moreno J, Krishnan AV, Feldman D. Molecular mechanisms mediating the anti-proliferative effects of Vitamin D in prostate cancer. *J Steroid Biochem Mol Biol,* 2005, 97: 31-36.

[11] Malloy PJ, Feldman D. Inactivation of the human vitamin D receptor by caspase-3. *Endocrinology*, 2009, 150: 679-686.

[12] Evans SR, Soldatenkov V, Shchepotin EB, Bogrash E, Shchepotin IB. Novel 19-nor-hexafluoride vitamin D_3 analog (Ro 25-6760) inhibits human colon cancer in vitro via apoptosis. *Int J Oncol*, 1999, 14: 979-985.

[13] Diaz GD, Paraskeva C, Thomas MG, Binderup L, Hague A. Apoptosis is induced by the active metabolite of vitamin D_3 and its analogue EB1089 in colorectal adenoma and carcinoma cells: possible implications for prevention and therapy. *Cancer Res*, 2000, 60: 2304-2312.

[14] Nittke T, Kallay E, Manhardt T, Cross HS. Parallel elevation of colonic 1,25-dihydroxyvitamin D_3 levels and apoptosis in female mice on a calcium-deficient diet. *Anticancer Res,* 2009, 29: 3727-3732.

[15] De Haes P, Garmyn M, Carmeliet G, Degreef H, Vantieghem K, Bouillon R, Segaert S. Molecular pathways involved in the anti-apoptotic effect of 1,25-dihydroxyvitamin D_3 in primary human keratinocytes. *J Cell Biochem*, 2004, 93: 951-967.

[16] Diker-Cohen T, Koren R, Ravid A. Programmed cell death of stressed keratinocytes and its inhibition by vitamin D: the role of death and survival signaling pathways. *Apoptosis*, 2006, 11: 519-534.

[17] Gupta R, Dixon KM, Deo SS, Holliday CJ, Slater M, Halliday GM, Reeve VE, Mason RS. Photoprotection by 1,25 dihydroxyvitamin D_3 is associated with an increase in p53 and a decrease in nitric oxide products. *J Invest Dermatol,* 2007, 127: 707-715.

[18] Langberg M, Rotem C, Fenig E, Koren R, Ravid A. Vitamin D protects keratinocytes from deleterious effects of ionizing radiation. *Br J Dermatol,* 2009, 160: 151-161.

[19] Duque G, El Abdaimi K, Henderson JE, Lomri A, Kremer R. Vitamin D inhibits Fas ligand-induced apoptosis in human osteoblasts by regulating components of both the mitochondrial and Fas-related pathways. *Bone*, 2004, 35: 57-64.

[20] Vertino AM, Bula CM, Chen JR, Almeida M, Han L, Bellido T, Kousteni S, Norman AW, Manolagas SC. Nongenotropic, anti-apoptotic signaling of 1alpha,25$(OH)_2$-vitamin D_3 and analogs through the ligand binding domain of the vitamin D receptor in osteoblasts and osteocytes. Mediation by Src, phosphatidylinositol 3-, and JNK kinases. *J Biol Chem,* 2005, 280: 14130-14137.

[21] Xiaoyu Z, Payal B, Melissa O, Zanello LP. 1alpha,25$(OH)_2$-vitamin D_3 membrane-initiated calcium signaling modulates exocytosis and cell survival. *J Steroid Biochem Mol Biol*, 2007, 103: 457-461.

[22] Zhang X, Zanello LP. Vitamin D receptor-dependent 1 alpha,25$(OH)_2$ vitamin D_3-induced anti-apoptotic PI3K/AKT signaling in osteoblasts. *J Bone Miner Res*, 2008, 23: 1238-1248.

[23] Xu HM, Tepper CG, Jones JB, Fernandez CE, Studzinski GP. 1,25-Dihydroxyvitamin D_3 protects HL60 cells against apoptosis but down-regulates the expression of the bcl-2 gene. *Exp Cell Res*, 1993, 209: 367-374.

[24] Wang X, Studzinski GP. Antiapoptotic action of 1,25-dihydroxyvitamin D_3 is associated with increased mitochondrial MCL-1 and RAF-1 proteins and reduced release of cytochrome c. *Exp Cell Res*, 1997, 235: 210-217.

[25] Wang X, Rao J, Studzinski GP. Inhibition of p38 MAP kinase activity up-regulates multiple MAP kinase pathways and potentiates 1,25-dihydroxyvitamin D_3-induced differentiation of human leukemia HL60 cells. *Exp Cell Res*, 2000, 258: 425-437.

[26] Wang X, Studzinski GP. Activation of extracellular signal-regulated kinases (ERKs) defines the first phase of 1,25-dihydroxyvitamin D_3-induced differentiation of HL60 cells. *J Cell Biochem,* 2001, 80: 471-482.

[27] Zhang Y, Zhang J, Studzinski GP. AKT pathway is activated by 1, 25-dihydroxyvitamin D_3 and participates in its anti-apoptotic effect and cell cycle control in differentiating HL60 cells. *Cell Cycle,* 2006, 5: 447-451.

[28] Wang X, Wang TT, White JH, Studzinski GP. Expression of human kinase suppressor of Ras 2 (hKSR-2) gene in HL60 leukemia cells is directly upregulated by 1,25-dihydroxyvitamin D_3 and is required for optimal cell differentiation. *Exp Cell Res,* 2007, 313: 3034-3045.

[29] Wang X, Patel R, Studzinski GP. hKSR-2, a vitamin D-regulated gene, inhibits apoptosis in arabinocytosine-treated HL60 leukemia cells. *Mol Cancer Ther*, 2008, 7: 2798-2806.

[30] Myrthue A, Rademacher BL, Pittsenbarger J, Kutyba-Brooks B, Gantner M, Qian DZ, Beer TM. The iroquois homeobox gene 5 is regulated by 1,25-dihydroxyvitamin D_3 in human prostate cancer and regulates apoptosis and the cell cycle in LNCaP prostate cancer cells. *Clin Cancer Res,* 2008, 14: 3562-3570.

[31] Simboli-Campbell M, Narvaez CJ, van Weelden K, Tenniswood M, Welsh J. Comparative effects of $1,25(OH)_2D_3$ and EB1089 on cell cycle kinetics and apoptosis in MCF-7 breast cancer cells. *Breast Cancer Res Treat,* 1997, 42: 31-41.

[32] Stewart LV, Weigel NL. Vitamin D and prostate cancer. *Exp Biol Med (*Maywood), 2004, 229: 277-284.

[33] Miyaura C, Abe E, Kuribayashi T, Tanaka H, Konno K, Nishii Y, Suda T. 1 alpha,25-Dihydroxyvitamin D_3 induces differentiation of human myeloid leukemia cells. *Biochem Biophys Res Commun*, 1981, 102: 937-943.

[34] Wang QM, Jones JB, Studzinski GP. Cyclin-dependent kinase inhibitor p27 as a mediator of the G1-S phase block induced by 1,25-dihydroxyvitamin D_3 in HL60 cells. *Cancer Res*, 1996, 56: 264-267.

[35] Campbell MJ, Elstner E, Holden S, Uskokovic M, Koeffler HP. Inhibition of proliferation of prostate cancer cells by a 19-nor-hexafluoride vitamin D_3 analogue involves the induction of $p21^{waf1}$, $p27^{kip1}$ and E-cadherin. *J Mol Endocrinol*, 1997, 19: 15-27.

[36] Park WH, Seol JG, Kim ES, Jung CW, Lee CC, Binderup L, Koeffler HP, Kim BK, Lee YY. Cell cycle arrest induced by the vitamin D_3 analog EB1089 in NCI-H929 myeloma cells is associated with induction of the cyclin-dependent kinase inhibitor p27. *Exp Cell Res*, 2000, 254: 279-286.

[37] Dackiw AP, Ezzat S, Huang P, Liu W, Asa SL. Vitamin D_3 administration induces nuclear p27 accumulation, restores

differentiation, and reduces tumor burden in a mouse model of metastatic follicular thyroid cancer. *Endocrinology*, 2004, 145: 5840-5846.

[38] Huang YC, Chen JY, Hung WC. Vitamin D_3 receptor/Sp1 complex is required for the induction of $p27^{Kip1}$ expression by vitamin D_3. *Oncogene*, 2004, 23: 4856-4861.

[39] Cheng HT, Chen JY, Huang YC, Chang HC, Hung WC. Functional role of VDR in the activation of $p27^{Kip1}$ by the VDR/Sp1 complex. *J Cell Biochem*, 2006, 98: 1450-1456.

[40] Lin R, Wang TT, Miller WH, Jr., White JH. Inhibition of F-Box protein p45(SKP2) expression and stabilization of cyclin-dependent kinase inhibitor p27(KIP1) in vitamin D analog-treated cancer cells. *Endocrinology*, 2003, 144: 749-753.

[41] Li P, Li C, Zhao X, Zhang X, Nicosia SV, Bai W. $p27^{Kip1}$ stabilization and G1 arrest by 1,25-dihydroxyvitamin D_3 in ovarian cancer cells mediated through down-regulation of cyclin E/cyclin-dependent kinase 2 and Skp1-Cullin-F-box protein/Skp2 ubiquitin ligase. *J Biol Chem*, 2004, 279: 25260-25267.

[42] Luo W, Chen Y, Liu M, Du K, Zheng G, Cai T, Zhang W, Zhao F, Yao T, Yang R, Chen J. EB1089 induces Skp2-dependent p27 accumulation, leading to cell growth inhibition and cell cycle G1 phase arrest in human hepatoma cells. *Cancer Invest,* 2009, 27: 29-37.

[43] Wang X, Gocek E, Liu CG, Studzinski GP. MicroRNAs181 regulate the expression of p27Kip1 in human myeloid leukemia cells induced to differentiate by 1,25-dihydroxyvitamin D_3. *Cell Cycle*, 2009, 8: 736-741.

[44] Jiang H, Lin J, Su ZZ, Collart FR, Huberman E, Fisher PB. Induction of differentiation in human promyelocytic HL-60 leukemia cells activates p21, WAF1/CIP1, expression in the absence of p53. *Oncogene*, 1994, 9: 3397-3406.

[45] Liu M, Lee MH, Cohen M, Bommakanti M, Freedman LP. Transcriptional activation of the Cdk inhibitor p21 by vitamin D_3 leads to the induced differentiation of the myelomonocytic cell line U937. *Genes Dev,* 1996, 10: 142-153.

[46] Verlinden L, Verstuyf A, Convents R, Marcelis S, Van Camp M, Bouillon R. Action of $1,25(OH)_2D_3$ on the cell cycle genes, cyclin D1, p21 and p27 in MCF-7 cells. *Mol Cell Endocrinol,* 1998, 142: 57-65.

[47] Gumireddy K, Reddy GS, Ikegaki N, Binderup L, Sutton LN, Phillips PC, Reddy CD. Anti-proliferative effects of 20-epi-vitamin-D_3 analogue,

KH1060 in human neuroblastoma: induction of RAR-beta and $p21^{Cip1}$. *Cancer Lett,* 2003, 190: 51-60.

[48] Moriwake T, Tanaka H, Kanzaki S, Higuchi J, Seino Y. 1,25-Dihydroxyvitamin D_3 stimulates the secretion of insulin-like growth factor binding protein 3 (IGFBP-3) by cultured human osteosarcoma cells. *Endocrinology*, 1992, 130: 1071-1073.

[49] Krishnan AV, Peehl DM, Feldman D. Inhibition of prostate cancer growth by vitamin D: Regulation of target gene expression. *J Cell Biochem*, 2003, 88: 363-371.

[50] Reichman TW, Albanell J, Wang X, Moore MA, Studzinski GP. Downregulation of telomerase activity in HL60 cells by differentiating agents is accompanied by increased expression of telomerase-associated protein. *J Cell Biochem*, 1997, 67: 13-23.

[51] Yamada O, Ozaki K, Nakatake M, Akiyama M, Kawauchi K, Matsuoka R. Multistep regulation of telomerase during differentiation of HL60 cells. *J Leukoc Biol*, 2008, 83: 1240-1248.

[52] Godyn JJ, Xu H, Zhang F, Kolla S, Studzinski GP. A dual block to cell cycle progression in HL60 cells exposed to analogues of vitamin D_3. *Cell Prolif*, 1994, 27: 37-46.

[53] Harrison LE, Wang QM, Studzinski GP. 1,25-dihydroxyvitamin D_3-induced retardation of the G_2/M traverse is associated with decreased levels of p34(cdc2) in HL60 cells. *J Cell Biochem*, 1999, 75: 226-234.

[54] Esquenet M, Swinnen JV, Heyns W, Verhoeven G. Control of LNCaP proliferation and differentiation: actions and interactions of androgens, 1alpha,25-dihydroxycholecalciferol, all-trans retinoic acid, 9-cis retinoic acid, and phenylacetate. *Prostate*, 1996, 28: 182-194.

[55] Zhao XY, Feldman D. The role of vitamin D in prostate cancer. *Steroids*, 2001, 66: 293-300.

[56] Beer TM, Garzotto M, Park B, Mori M, Myrthue A, Janeba N, Sauer D, Eilers K. Effect of calcitriol on prostate-specific antigen in vitro and in humans. *Clin Cancer Res,* 2006, 12: 2812-2816.

[57] Agadir A, Lazzaro G, Zheng Y, Zhang XK, Mehta R. Resistance of HBL100 human breast epithelial cells to vitamin D action. *Carcinogenesis*, 1999, 20: 577-582.

[58] Wang Q, Lee D, Sysounthone V, Chandraratna RAS, Christakos S, Korah R, Wieder R. 1,25-dihydroxyvitamin D_3 and retinoic acid analogues induce differentiation in breast cancer cells with function- and cell-specific additive effects. *Breast Cancer Res Treat,* 2001, 67: 157-168.

[59] Welsh J. Vitamin D and breast cancer: insights from animal models. *Am J Clin Nutr,* 2004, 80: 1721S-1724S.

[60] Pendas-Franco N, Gonzalez-Sancho JM, Suarez Y, Aguilera O, Steinmeyer A, Gamallo C, Berciano MT, Lafarga M, Munoz A. Vitamin D regulates the phenotype of human breast cancer cells. *Differentiation*, 2007, 75: 193-207.

[61] Garland CF, Comstock GW, Garland FC, Helsing KJ, Shaw EK, Gorham ED. Serum 25-hydroxyvitamin D and colon cancer: eight-year prospective study. *Lancet*, 1989, 2: 1176-1178.

[62] Chen A, Davis BH, Bissonnette M, Scaglione-Sewell B, Brasitus TA. 1,25-Dihydroxyvitamin D_3 stimulates activator protein-1-dependent Caco-2 cell differentiation. *J Biol Chem,* 1999, 274: 35505-35513.

[63] Palmer HG, Sanchez-Carbayo M, Ordonez-Moran P, Larriba MJ, Cordon-Cardo C, Munoz A. Genetic signatures of differentiation induced by 1alpha,25-dihydroxyvitamin D_3 in human colon cancer cells. *Cancer Res*, 2003, 63: 7799-7806.

[64] Aguilera O, Pena C, Garcia JM, Larriba MJ, Ordonez-Moran P, Navarro D, Barbachano A, Lopez de Silanes I, Ballestar E, Fraga MF, Esteller M, Gamallo C, Bonilla F, Gonzalez-Sancho JM, Munoz A. The Wnt antagonist DICKKOPF-1 gene is induced by 1alpha,25-dihydroxyvitamin D_3 associated to the differentiation of human colon cancer cells. *Carcinogenesis*, 2007, 28: 1877-1884.

[65] Giovannucci E, Liu Y, Rimm EB, Hollis BW, Fuchs CS, Stampfer MJ, Willett WC. Prospective study of predictors of vitamin D status and cancer incidence and mortality in men. *J Natl Cancer Inst*, 2006, 98: 451-459.

[66] Moore TB, Sidell N, Chow VJ, Medzoyan RH, Huang JI, Yamashiro JM, Wada RK. Differentiating effects of 1,25-dihydroxycholecalciferol D_3 on LA-N-5 human neuroblastoma cells and its synergy with retinoic acid. *J Pediatr Hematol Oncol,* 1995, 17: 311-317.

[67] Abe E, Miyaura C, Sakagami H, Takeda M, Konno K, Yamazaki T, Yoshiki S, Suda T. *Differentiation of mouse myeloid leukemia cells induced by 1 alpha,25-dihydroxyvitamin* D_3. Proc Natl Acad Sci U S A, 1981, 78: 4990-4994.

[68] Bunce CM, French PJ, Durham J, Stockley RA, Michell RH, Brown G. Indomethacin potentiates the induction of HL60 differentiation to neutrophils, by retinoic acid and granulocyte colony-stimulating factor, and to monocytes, by vitamin D_3. *Leukemia*, 1994, 8: 595-604.

[69] Hughes PJ, Brown G. 1alpha,25-dihydroxyvitamin D_3-mediated stimulation of steroid sulphatase activity in myeloid leukaemic cell lines requires VDRnuc-mediated activation of the RAS/RAF/ERK-MAP kinase signalling pathway. *J Cell Biochem*, 2006, 98: 590-617.

[70] Hughes PJ, Lee JS, Reiner NE, Brown G. The vitamin D receptor-mediated activation of phosphatidylinositol 3-kinase (PI3Kalpha) plays a role in the 1alpha,25-dihydroxyvitamin D_3-stimulated increase in steroid sulphatase activity in myeloid leukaemic cell lines. *J Cell Biochem,* 2008, 103: 1551-1572.

[71] Marcinkowska E, Wiedlocha A, Radzikowski C. 1,25-Dihydroxyvitamin D_3 induced activation and subsequent nuclear translocation of MAPK is upstream regulated by PKC in HL-60 cells. *Biochem Biophys Res Commun,* 1997, 241: 419-426.

[72] Marcinkowska E. Evidence that activation of MEK1,2/erk1,2 signal transduction pathway is necessary for calcitriol-induced differentiation of HL-60 cells. *Anticancer Res,* 2001, 21: 499-504.

[73] Mangelsdorf DJ, Koeffler HP, Donaldson CA, Pike JW, Haussler MR. 1,25-Dihydroxyvitamin D_3-induced differentiation in a human promyelocytic leukemia cell line (HL-60): receptor-mediated maturation to macrophage-like cells. *J Cell Biol,* 1984, 98: 391-398.

[74] Studzinski GP, Bhandal AK, Brelvi ZS. A system for monocytic differentiation of leukemic cells HL 60 by a short exposure to 1,25-dihydroxycholecalciferol. *Proc Soc Exp Biol Med*, 1985, 179: 288-295.

[75] Perkins SL, Link DC, Kling S, Ley TJ, Teitelbaum SL. 1,25-Dihydroxyvitamin D_3 induces monocytic differentiation of the PLB-985 leukemic line and promotes c-fgr mRNA expression. *J Leukoc Biol*, 1991, 50: 427-433.

[76] Rao DS, Campbell MJ, Koeffler HP, Ishizuka S, Uskokovic MR, Spagnuolo P, Reddy GS. Metabolism of 1alpha,25-dihydroxyvitamin D_3 in human promyelocytic leukemia (HL-60) cells: in vitro biological activities of the natural metabolites of 1alpha,25-dihydroxyvitamin D_3 produced in HL-60 cells. *Steroids*, 2001, 66: 423-431.

[77] Munker R, Kobayashi T, Elstner E, Norman AW, Uskokovic M, Zhang W, Andreeff M, Koeffler HP. A new series of vitamin D analogs is highly active for clonal inhibition, differentiation, and induction of WAF1 in myeloid leukemia. *Blood*, 1996, 88: 2201-2209.

[78] Wang Q, Wang X, Studzinski GP. Jun N-terminal kinase pathway enhances signaling of monocytic differentiation of human leukemia cells

induced by 1,25-dihydroxyvitamin D_3. *J Cell Biochem*, 2003, 89: 1087-1101.

[79] Wang X, Studzinski GP. Inhibition of p38MAP kinase potentiates the JNK/SAPK pathway and AP-1 activity in monocytic but not in macrophage or granulocytic differentiation of HL60 cells. *J Cell Biochem,* 2001, 82: 68-77.

[80] Chen-Deutsch X, Garay E, Zhang J, Harrison JS, Studzinski GP. c-Jun N-terminal kinase 2 (JNK2) antagonizes the signaling of differentiation by JNK1 in human myeloid leukemia cells resistant to vitamin D. *Leuk Res*, 2009, 33: 1372-1378.

[81] Wang X, Studzinski GP. Raf-1 signaling is required for the later stages of 1,25-dihydroxyvitamin D_3-induced differentiation of HL60 cells but is not mediated by the MEK/ERK module. J Cell Physiol, 2006, 209: 253-260.

[82] Jamshidi F, Zhang J, Harrison JS, Wang X, Studzinski GP. Induction of differentiation of human leukemia cells by combinations of COX inhibitors and 1,25-dihydroxyvitamin D_3 involves Raf1 but not Erk 1/2 signaling. *Cell Cycle*, 2008, 7: 917-924.

[83] Wang X, Studzinski GP. Phosphorylation of raf-1 by kinase suppressor of ras is inhibited by "MEK-specific" inhibitors PD 098059 and U0126 in differentiating HL60 cells. *Exp Cell Res,* 2001, 268: 294-300.

[84] Wang X, Studzinski GP. Kinase suppressor of RAS (KSR) amplifies the differentiation signal provided by low concentrations 1,25-dihydroxyvitamin D_3. *J Cell Physiol,* 2004, 198: 333-342.

[85] Wang X, Wang TT, White JH, Studzinski GP. Induction of kinase suppressor of RAS-1(KSR-1) gene by 1, alpha25-dihydroxyvitamin D_3 in human leukemia HL60 cells through a vitamin D response element in the 5'-flanking region. *Oncogene*, 2006, 25: 7078-7085.

[86] Wang X, Studzinski GP. The requirement for and changing composition of the activating protein-1 transcription factor during differentiation of human leukemia HL60 cells induced by 1,25-dihydroxyvitamin D_3. *Cancer Res,* 2006, 66: 4402-4409.

[87] Ji Y, Studzinski GP. Retinoblastoma protein and CCAAT/enhancer-binding protein beta are required for 1,25-dihydroxyvitamin D_3-induced monocytic differentiation of HL60 cells. *Cancer Res,* 2004, 64: 370-377.

[88] Marcinkowska E, Garay E, Gocek E, Chrobak A, Wang X, Studzinski GP. Regulation of C/EBPbeta isoforms by MAPK pathways in HL60 cells induced to differentiate by 1,25-dihydroxyvitamin D_3. *Exp Cell Res,* 2006, 312: 2054-2065.

[89] Koschmieder S, Agrawal S, Radomska HS, Huettner CS, Tenen DG, Ottmann OG, Berdel WE, Serve HL, Muller-Tidow C. Decitabine and vitamin D_3 differentially affect hematopoietic transcription factors to induce monocytic differentiation. *Int J Oncol,* 2007, 30: 349-355.
[90] Moeenrezakhanlou A, Shephard L, Lam L, Reiner NE. Myeloid cell differentiation in response to calcitriol for expression CD11b and CD14 is regulated by myeloid zinc finger-1 protein downstream of phosphatidylinositol 3-kinase. *J Leukoc Biol,* 2008, 84: 519-528.
[91] Pahl HL, Scheibe RJ, Zhang DE, Chen HM, Galson DL, Maki RA, Tenen DG. The proto-oncogene PU.1 regulates expression of the myeloid-specific CD11b promoter. *J Biol Chem,* 1993, 268: 5014-5020.
[92] Pan Z, Hetherington CJ, Zhang DE. CCAAT/enhancer-binding protein activates the CD14 promoter and mediates transforming growth factor beta signaling in monocyte development. *J Biol Chem*, 1999, 274: 23242-23248.
[93] Zhang F, Godyn JJ, Uskokovic M, Binderup L, Studzinski GP. Monocytic differentiation of HL60 cells induced by potent analogs of vitamin D_3 precedes the G1/G0 phase cell cycle block. *Cell Proliferation*, 1994, 27: 643-654.
[94] Studzinski GP, Rathod B, Wang QM, Rao J, Zhang F. Uncoupling of cell cycle arrest from the expression of monocytic differentiation markers in HL60 cell variants. *Exp Cell Res*, 1997, 232: 376-387.
[95] Studzinski GP, Bhandal AK, Brelvi ZS. Cell cycle sensitivity of HL-60 cells to the differentiation-inducing effects of 1-alpha,25-dihydroxyvitamin D_3. *Cancer Res,* 1985, 45: 3898-3905.
[96] Chen F, Studzinski GP. Cyclin-dependent kinase 5 activity enhances monocytic phenotype and cell cycle traverse in 1,25-dihydroxyvitamin D_3-treated HL60 cells. *Exp Cell Res,* 1999, 249: 422-428.
[97] Chen F, Rao J, Studzinski GP. Specific association of increased cyclin-dependent kinase 5 expression with monocytic lineage of differentiation of human leukemia HL60 cells. *J Leukoc Biol,* 2000, 67: 559-566.
[98] Chen F, Wang Q, Wang X, Studzinski GP. Up-regulation of Egr1 by 1,25-dihydroxyvitamin D_3 contributes to increased expression of p35 activator of cyclin-dependent kinase 5 and consequent onset of the terminal phase of HL60 cell differentiation. *Cancer Res,* 2004, 64: 5425-5433.
[99] Studzinski GP, Wang X, Ji Y, Wang Q, Zhang Y, Kutner A, Harrison JS. The rationale for deltanoids in therapy for myeloid leukemia: role of

KSR-MAPK-C/EBP pathway. *J Steroid Biochem Mol Biol*, 2005, 97: 47-55.

[100] Zhang J, Harrison JS, Uskokovic M, Danilenko M, Studzinski GP. Silibinin can induce differentiation as well as enhance vitamin D_3-induced differentiation of human AML cells ex vivo and regulates the levels of differentiation-related transcription factors. *Hematol Oncol,* 2009, 27: (in press).

[101] Potter GK, Mohamed AN, Dracopoli NC, Groshen SL, Shen RN, Moore MA. Action of 1,25-$(OH)_2D_3$ in nude mice bearing transplantable human myelogenous leukemic cell lines. *Exp Hematol,* 1985, 13: 722-732.

[102] Eisman JA, Barkla DH, Tutton PJ. Suppression of in vivo growth of human cancer solid tumor xenografts by 1,25-dihydroxyvitamin D_3. *Cancer Res*, 1987, 47: 21-25.

[103] Hershberger PA, Modzelewski RA, Shurin ZR, Rueger RM, Trump DL, Johnson CS. 1,25-Dihydroxycholecalciferol (1,25-D_3) inhibits the growth of squamous cell carcinoma and down-modulates $p21^{Waf1/Cip1}$ in vitro and in vivo. *Cancer Res*, 1999, 59: 2644-2649.

[104] Pourgholami MH, Akhter J, Lu Y, Morris DL. In vitro and in vivo inhibition of liver cancer cells by 1,25-dihydroxyvitamin D_3. *Cancer Lett*, 2000, 151: 97-102.

[105] Banach-Petrosky W, Ouyang X, Gao H, Nader K, Ji Y, Suh N, DiPaola RS, Abate-Shen C. Vitamin D inhibits the formation of prostatic intraepithelial neoplasia in Nkx3.1;Pten mutant mice. *Clin Cancer Res*, 2006, 12: 5895-5901.

[106] Koeffler HP, Hirji K, Itri L. 1,25-Dihydroxyvitamin D_3: in vivo and in vitro effects on human preleukemic and leukemic cells. *Cancer Treat Rep,* 1985, 69: 1399-1407.

[107] Osborn JL, Schwartz GG, Smith DC, Bahnson R, Day R, Trump DL. Phase II Trial of Oral 1,25-Dihydroxyvitamin D (Calcitriol) in Hormone Refractory Prostate Cancer. *Urologic Oncology: Seminars and Original Investigations*, 1995, 1: 195-198.

[108] Beer TM, Javle MM, Ryan CW, Garzotto M, Lam GN, Wong A, Henner WD, Johnson CS, Trump DL. Phase I study of weekly DN-101, a new formulation of calcitriol, in patients with cancer. *Cancer Chemother Pharmacol,* 2007, 59: 581-587.

[109] Trump DL, Hershberger PA, Bernardi RJ, Ahmed S, Muindi J, Fakih M, Yu WD, Johnson CS. Anti-tumor activity of calcitriol: pre-clinical and clinical studies. *J Steroid Biochem Mol Biol,* 2004, 89-90: 519-526.

[110] Srinivas S, Feldman D. A phase II trial of calcitriol and naproxen in recurrent prostate cancer. *Anticancer Res*, 2009, 29: 3605-3610.

[111] Tiffany NM, Ryan CW, Garzotto M, Wersinger EM, Beer TM. High dose pulse calcitriol, docetaxel and estramustine for androgen independent prostate cancer: a phase I/II study. *J Urol,* 2005, 174: 888-892.

[112] Flaig TW, Barqawi A, Miller G, Kane M, Zeng C, Crawford ED, Glode LM. A phase II trial of dexamethasone, vitamin D, and carboplatin in patients with hormone-refractory prostate cancer. *Cancer*, 2006, 107: 266-274.

[113] Beer TM, Ryan CW, Venner PM, Petrylak DP, Chatta GS, Ruether JD, Redfern CH, Fehrenbacher L, Saleh MN, Waterhouse DM, Carducci MA, Vicario D, Dreicer R, Higano CS, Ahmann FR, Chi KN, Henner WD, Arroyo A, Clow FW. Double-blinded randomized study of high-dose calcitriol plus docetaxel compared with placebo plus docetaxel in androgen-independent prostate cancer: a report from the ASCENT Investigators. *J Clin Oncol,* 2007, 25: 669-674.

[114] Schwartz GG. Vitamin D and intervention trials in prostate cancer: from theory to therapy. *Ann Epidemiol,* 2009, 19: 96-102.

[115] Eelen G, Gysemans C, Verlinden L, Vanoirbeek E, De Clercq P, Van Haver D, Mathieu C, Bouillon R, Verstuyf A. Mechanism and potential of the growth-inhibitory actions of vitamin D and analogs. *Curr Med Chem,* 2007, 14: 1893-1910.

[116] Brown AJ, Slatopolsky E. Vitamin D analogs: therapeutic applications and mechanisms for selectivity. *Mol Aspects Med,* 2008, 29: 433-452.

[117] Binderup L, Bramm E. Effects of a novel vitamin D analogue MC903 on cell proliferation and differentiation in vitro and on calcium metabolism in vivo. *Biochem Pharmacol,* 1988, 37: 889-895.

[118] Colston KW, Mackay AG, James SY, Binderup L, Chander S, Coombes RC. EB1089: a new vitamin D analogue that inhibits the growth of breast cancer cells in vivo and in vitro. *Biochem Pharmacol*, 1992, 44: 2273-2280.

[119] Valrance ME, Brunet AH, Welsh J. Vitamin D receptor-dependent inhibition of mammary tumor growth by EB1089 and ultraviolet radiation in vivo. *Endocrinology*, 2007, 148: 4887-4894.

[120] Kawa S, Yoshizawa K, Nikaido T, Kiyosawa K. Inhibitory effect of 22-oxa-1,25-dihydroxyvitamin D_3, maxacalcitol, on the proliferation of pancreatic cancer cell lines. *J Steroid Biochem Mol Biol*, 2005, 97: 173-177.

[121] Binderup L, Latini S, Binderup E, Bretting C, Calverley M, Hansen K. 20-epi-vitamin D_3 analogues: a novel class of potent regulators of cell growth and immune responses. *Biochem Pharmacol,* 1991, 42: 1569-1575.

[122] Norman AW, Manchand PS, Uskokovic MR, Okamura WH, Takeuchi JA, Bishop JE, Hisatake JI, Koeffler HP, Peleg S. Characterization of a novel analogue of 1alpha,25$(OH)_2$-vitamin D_3 with two side chains: interaction with its nuclear receptor and cellular actions. *J Med Chem,* 2000, 43: 2719-2730.

[123] O'Kelly J, Uskokovic M, Lemp N, Vadgama J, Koeffler HP. Novel Gemini-vitamin D_3 analog inhibits tumor cell growth and modulates the Akt/mTOR signaling pathway. *J Steroid Biochem Mol Biol,* 2006, 100: 107-116.

[124] Garay E, Jankowski P, Lizano P, Marczak S, Maehr H, Adorini L, Uskokovic MR, Studzinski GP. Calcitriol derivatives with two different side-chains at C-20. Part 4: further chain modifications that alter VDR-dependent monocytic differentiation potency in human leukemia cells. *Bioorg Med Chem*, 2007, 15: 4444-4455.

[125] Saito T, Okamoto R, Haritunians T, O'Kelly J, Uskokovic M, Maehr H, Marczak S, Jankowski P, Badr R, Koeffler HP. Novel Gemini vitamin D_3 analogs have potent antitumor activity. *J Steroid Biochem Mol Biol,* 2008, 112: 151-156.

[126] Maehr H, Lee HJ, Perry B, Suh N, Uskokovic MR. Calcitriol Derivatives with Two Different Side Chains at C-20. V. Potent Inhibitors of Mammary Carcinogenesis and Inducers of Leukemia Differentiation (dagger). *J Med Chem*, 2009.

[127] Posner GH, Lee JK, Wang Q, Peleg S, Burke M, Brem H, Dolan P, Kensler TW. Noncalcemic, antiproliferative, transcriptionally active, 24-fluorinated hybrid analogues of the hormone 1alpha, 25-dihydroxyvitamin D_3. Synthesis and preliminary biological evaluation. *J Med Chem*, 1998, 41: 3008-3014.

[128] Alagbala AA, Johnson CS, Trump DL, Posner GH, Foster BA. Antitumor effects of two less-calcemic vitamin D analogs (Paricalcitol and QW-1624F2-2) in squamous cell carcinoma cells. *Oncology*, 2006, 70: 483-492.

[129] Zhang J, Posner GH, Danilenko M, Studzinski GP. Differentiation-inducing potency of the seco-steroid JK-1624F2-2 can be increased by combination with an antioxidant and a p38MAPK inhibitor which

upregulates the JNK pathway. *J Steroid Biochem Mol Biol,* 2007, 105: 140-149.

[130] Mehta RG, Moriarty RM, Mehta RR, Penmasta R, Lazzaro G, Constantinou A, Guo L. Prevention of preneoplastic mammary lesion development by a novel vitamin D analogue, 1alpha-hydroxyvitamin D_5. *J Natl Cancer Inst,* 1997, 89: 212-218.

[131] Hussain-Hakimjee EA, Peng X, Mehta RR, Mehta RG. Growth inhibition of carcinogen-transformed MCF-12F breast epithelial cells and hormone-sensitive BT-474 breast cancer cells by 1alpha-hydroxyvitamin D_5. *Carcinogenesis*, 2006, 27: 551-559.

[132] Luong QT, Koeffler HP. Vitamin D compounds in leukemia. *J Steroid Biochem Mol Biol,* 2005, 97: 195-202.

[133] Vijayakumar S, Mehta RR, Boerner PS, Packianathan S, Mehta RG. Clinical trials involving vitamin D analogs in prostate cancer. *Cancer J,* 2005, 11: 362-373.

[134] Vijayakumar S, Boerner PS, Mehta RR, Packianathan S, Mehta RG, Das Gupta TK. Clinical trials using chemopreventive vitamin D analogs in breast cancer. *Cancer J,* 2006, 12: 445-450.

[135] Masuda S, Jones G. Promise of vitamin D analogues in the treatment of hyperproliferative conditions. *Mol Cancer Ther,* 2006, 5: 797-808.

[136] Evans TR, Colston KW, Lofts FJ, Cunningham D, Anthoney DA, Gogas H, de Bono JS, Hamberg KJ, Skov T, Mansi JL. A phase II trial of the vitamin D analogue Seocalcitol (EB1089) in patients with inoperable pancreatic cancer. *Br J Cancer,* 2002, 86: 680-685.

[137] Gulliford T, English J, Colston KW, Menday P, Moller S, Coombes RC. A phase I study of the vitamin D analogue EB 1089 in patients with advanced breast and colorectal cancer. *Br J Cancer*, 1998, 78: 6-13.

[138] Dalhoff K, Dancey J, Astrup L, Skovsgaard T, Hamberg KJ, Lofts FJ, Rosmorduc O, Erlinger S, Bach Hansen J, Steward WP, Skov T, Burcharth F, Evans TR. A phase II study of the vitamin D analogue Seocalcitol in patients with inoperable hepatocellular carcinoma. *Br J Cancer*, 2003, 89: 252-257.

[139] Koeffler HP, Aslanian N, O'Kelly J. Vitamin D_2 analog (Paricalcitol; Zemplar) for treatment of myelodysplastic syndrome. *Leuk Res*, 2005, 29: 1259-1262.

[140] Petrich A, Kahl B, Bailey H, Kim K, Turman N, Juckett M. Phase II study of doxercalciferol for the treatment of myelodysplastic syndrome. *Leuk Lymphoma,* 2008, 49: 57-61.

[141] Liu G, Wilding G, Staab MJ, Horvath D, Miller K, Dresen A, Alberti D, Arzoomanian R, Chappell R, Bailey HH. Phase II study of 1alpha-hydroxyvitamin D_2 in the treatment of advanced androgen-independent prostate cancer. *Clin Cancer Res,* 2003, 9: 4077-4083.
[142] Schwartz GG, Hall MC, Stindt D, Patton S, Lovato J, Torti FM. Phase I/II study of 19-nor-1alpha-25-dihydroxyvitamin D_2 (paricalcitol) in advanced, androgen-insensitive prostate cancer. *Clin Cancer Res,* 2005, 11: 8680-8685.
[143] Attia S, Eickhoff J, Wilding G, McNeel D, Blank J, Ahuja H, Jumonville A, Eastman M, Shevrin D, Glode M, Alberti D, Staab MJ, Horvath D, Straus J, Marnocha R, Liu G. Randomized, double-blinded phase II evaluation of docetaxel with or without doxercalciferol in patients with metastatic, androgen-independent prostate cancer. *Clin Cancer Res,* 2008, 14: 2437-2443.
[144] Colli E, Rigatti P, Montorsi F, Artibani W, Petta S, Mondaini N, Scarpa R, Usai P, Olivieri L, Maggi M. BXL628, a novel vitamin D_3 analog arrests prostate growth in patients with benign prostatic hyperplasia: a randomized clinical trial. *Eur Urol*, 2006, 49: 82-86.
[145] Miyaura C, Abe E, Honma Y, Hozumi M, Nishii Y, Suda T. Cooperative effect of 1 alpha,25-dihydroxyvitamin D_3 and dexamethasone in inducing differentiation of mouse myeloid leukemia cells. *Arch Biochem Biophys,* 1983, 227: 379-385.
[146] Olsson I, Gullberg U, Ivhed I, Nilsson K. Induction of differentiation of the human histiocytic lymphoma cell line U-937 by 1 alpha,25-dihydroxycholecalciferol. *Cancer Res*, 1983, 43: 5862-5867.
[147] Danilenko M, Studzinski GP. Enhancement by other compounds of the anti-cancer activity of vitamin D_3 and its analogs. *Exp Cell Res*, 2004, 298: 339-358.
[148] Peehl DM, Feldman D. Interaction of nuclear receptor ligands with the Vitamin D signaling pathway in prostate cancer. *J Steroid Biochem Mol Biol,* 2004, 92: 307-315.
[149] Swami S, Krishnan AV, Moreno J, Bhattacharyya RB, Peehl DM, Feldman D. Calcitriol and genistein actions to inhibit the prostaglandin pathway: potential combination therapy to treat prostate cancer. *J Nutr,* 2007, 137: 205S-210S.
[150] Jurutka PW, Bartik L, Whitfield GK, Mathern DR, Barthel TK, Gurevich M, Hsieh JC, Kaczmarska M, Haussler CA, Haussler MR. Vitamin D receptor: key roles in bone mineral pathophysiology,

molecular mechanism of action, and novel nutritional ligands. *J Bone Miner Res,* 2007, 22 Suppl 2: V2-10.

[151] James SY, Williams MA, Newland AC, Colston KW. Leukemia cell differentiation: cellular and molecular interactions of retinoids and vitamin D. *Gen Pharmacol*, 1999, 32: 143-154.

[152] Mernitz H, Smith DE, Wood RJ, Russell RM, Wang XD. Inhibition of lung carcinogenesis by 1alpha,25-dihydroxyvitamin D_3 and 9-cis retinoic acid in the A/J mouse model: evidence of retinoid mitigation of vitamin D toxicity. *Int J Cancer*, 2007, 120: 1402-1409.

[153] Bhatia M, Kirkland JB, Meckling-Gill KA. M-CSF and 1,25-dihydroxyvitamin D_3 synergize with 12-O-tetradecanoylphorbol-13-acetate to induce macrophage differentiation in acute promyelocytic leukemia NB4 cells. *Leukemia*, 1994, 8: 1744-1749.

[154] Shimizu T, Kuromi A, Takeda K. Synergistic induction of gene expression during the differentiation into mature macrophage in human myeloblastic leukemia cells treated with TPA and KH1060. *Leuk Res,* 2009, 33: 803-809.

[155] Song XD, Norman AW. Bryostatin-1 and 1alpha,25-dihydroxyvitamin D_3 synergistically stimulate the differentiation of NB4 acute promyelocytic leukemia cells. *Leukemia*, 1999, 13: 275-281.

[156] Studzinski GP, Reddy KB, Hill HZ, Bhandal AK. Potentiation of 1-beta-D-arabinofuranosylcytosine cytotoxicity to HL-60 cells by 1,25-dihydroxyvitamin D_3 correlates with reduced rate of maturation of DNA replication intermediates. *Cancer Res*, 1991, 51: 3451-3455.

[157] Ma Y, Yu WD, Hershberger PA, Flynn G, Kong RX, Trump DL, Johnson CS. 1alpha,25-Dihydroxyvitamin D_3 potentiates cisplatin antitumor activity by p73 induction in a squamous cell carcinoma model. *Mol Cancer Ther*, 2008, 7: 3047-3055.

[158] Ting HJ, Hsu J, Bao BY, Lee YF. Docetaxel-induced growth inhibition and apoptosis in androgen independent prostate cancer cells are enhanced by 1alpha,25-dihydroxyvitamin D_3. *Cancer Lett,* 2007, 247: 122-129.

[159] Young MR, Lathers DM. Combination docetaxel plus vitamin D_3 as an immune therapy in animals bearing squamous cell carcinomas. *Otolaryngol Head Neck Surg*, 2005, 133: 611-618.

[160] Pelczynska M, Switalska M, Maciejewska M, Jaroszewicz I, Kutner A, Opolski A. Antiproliferative activity of vitamin D compounds in combination with cytostatics. *Anticancer Res*, 2006, 26: 2701-2705.

[161] Wietrzyk J, Milczarek M, Kutner A. The effect of combined treatment on head and neck human cancer cell lines with novel analogs of calcitriol and cytostatics. *Oncol Res*, 2007, 16: 517-525.
[162] Kumagai T, Shih LY, Hughes SV, Desmond JC, O'Kelly J, Hewison M, Koeffler HP. 19-Nor-1,25$(OH)_2D_2$ (a novel, noncalcemic vitamin D analogue), combined with arsenic trioxide, has potent antitumor activity against myeloid leukemia. *Cancer Res,* 2005, 65: 2488-2497.
[163] Koren R, Wacksberg S, Weitsman GE, Ravid A. Calcitriol sensitizes colon cancer cells to H_2O_2-induced cytotoxicity while inhibiting caspase activation. *J Steroid Biochem Mol Biol,* 2006, 101: 151-160.
[164] Marchionatti AM, Picotto G, Narvaez CJ, Welsh J, Tolosa de Talamoni NG. Antiproliferative action of menadione and 1,25$(OH)_2D_3$ on breast cancer cells. *J Steroid Biochem Mol Biol*, 2009, 113: 227-232.
[165] DeMasters GA, Gupta MS, Jones KR, Cabot M, Wang H, Gennings C, Park M, Bratland A, Ree AH, Gewirtz DA. Potentiation of cell killing by fractionated radiation and suppression of proliferative recovery in MCF-7 breast tumor cells by the Vitamin D_3 analog EB 1089. *J Steroid Biochem Mol Biol,* 2004, 92: 365-374.
[166] Niitsu N, Hayashi Y, Sugita K, Honma Y. Sensitization by 5-aza-2'-deoxycytidine of leukaemia cells with MLL abnormalities to induction of differentiation by all-trans retinoic acid and 1alpha,25-dihydroxyvitamin D_3. Br *J Haematol,* 2001, 112: 315-326.
[167] Hoessly MC, Rossi RM, Fischkoff SA. Factors responsible for variable reported lineages of HL-60 cells induced to mature with butyric acid. *Cancer Res*, 1989, 49: 3594-3597.
[168] Rashid SF, Moore JS, Walker E, Driver PM, Engel J, Edwards CE, Brown G, Uskokovic MR, Campbell MJ. Synergistic growth inhibition of prostate cancer cells by 1alpha,25 Dihydroxyvitamin D_3 and its 19-nor-hexafluoride analogs in combination with either sodium butyrate or trichostatin A. *Oncogene*, 2001, 20: 1860-1872.
[169] Malinen M, Saramaki A, Ropponen A, Degenhardt T, Vaisanen S, Carlberg C. Distinct HDACs regulate the transcriptional response of human cyclin-dependent kinase inhibitor genes to Trichostatin A and 1alpha,25-dihydroxyvitamin D_3. *Nucleic Acids Res*, 2008, 36: 121-132.
[170] Abedin SA, Banwell CM, Colston KW, Carlberg C, Campbell MJ. Epigenetic corruption of VDR signalling in malignancy. *Anticancer Res,* 2006, 26: 2557-2566.
[171] Krishnan AV, Moreno J, Nonn L, Swami S, Peehl DM, Feldman D. Calcitriol as a chemopreventive and therapeutic agent in prostate cancer:

role of anti-inflammatory activity. *J Bone Miner Res*, 2007, 22 Suppl 2: V74-80.

[172] Laverny G, Penna G, Uskokovic M, Marczak S, Maehr H, Jankowski P, Ceailles C, Vouros P, Smith B, Robinson M, Reddy GS, Adorini L. Synthesis and anti-inflammatory properties of 1alpha,25-dihydroxy-16-ene-20-cyclopropyl-24-oxo-vitamin D_3, a hypocalcemic, stable metabolite of 1alpha,25-dihydroxy-16-ene-20-cyclopropyl-vitamin D_3. *J Med Chem,* 2009, 52: 2204-2213.

[173] Gavrilov V, Steiner M, Shany S. The combined treatment of 1,25-dihydroxyvitamin D_3 and a non-steroid anti-inflammatory drug is highly effective in suppressing prostate cancer cell line (LNCaP) growth. *Anticancer Res*, 2005, 25: 3425-3429.

[174] Moreno J, Krishnan AV, Swami S, Nonn L, Peehl DM, Feldman D. Regulation of prostaglandin metabolism by calcitriol attenuates growth stimulation in prostate cancer cells. *Cancer Res*, 2005, 65: 7917-7925.

[175] Sokoloski JA, Sartorelli AC. Induction of the differentiation of HL-60 promyelocytic leukemia cells by nonsteroidal anti-inflammatory agents in combination with low levels of vitamin D_3. *Leuk-Res*, 1998, 22: 153-161.

[176] Kaler P, Augenlicht L, Klampfer L. Macrophage-derived IL-1beta stimulates Wnt signaling and growth of colon cancer cells: a crosstalk interrupted by vitamin D_3. *Oncogene*, 2009.

[177] Weitsman GE, Ravid A, Liberman UA, Koren R. The role of p38 MAP kinase in the synergistic cytotoxic action of calcitriol and TNF-alpha in human breast cancer cells. *J Steroid Biochem Mol Biol,* 2004, 89-90: 361-364.

[178] Golovko O, Nazarova N, Tuohimaa P. Vitamin D-induced up-regulation of tumour necrosis factor alpha (TNF-alpha) in prostate cancer cells. *Life Sci,* 2005, 77: 562-577.

[179] Wang X, Gardner JP, Kheir A, Uskokovic MR, Studzinski GP. Synergistic induction of HL60 cell differentiation by ketoconazole and 1-desoxy analogues of vitamin D_3. *J Natl Cancer Inst,* 1997, 89: 1199-1206.

[180] Peehl DM, Seto E, Hsu JY, Feldman D. Preclinical activity of ketoconazole in combination with calcitriol or the vitamin D analogue EB 1089 in prostate cancer cells. *J Urol,* 2002, 168: 1583-1588.

[181] Yee SW, Campbell MJ, Simons C. Inhibition of Vitamin D_3 metabolism enhances VDR signalling in androgen-independent prostate cancer cells. *J Steroid Biochem Mol Biol*, 2006, 98: 228-235.

[182] Lou YR, Tuohimaa P. Androgen enhances the antiproliferative activity of vitamin D_3 by suppressing 24-hydroxylase expression in LNCaP cells. *J Steroid Biochem Mol Biol,* 2006, 99: 44-49.

[183] Ikezoe T, Bandobashi K, Yang Y, Takeuchi S, Sekiguchi N, Sakai S, Koeffler HP, Taguchi H. HIV-1 protease inhibitor ritonavir potentiates the effect of 1,25-dihydroxyvitamin D_3 to induce growth arrest and differentiation of human myeloid leukemia cells via down-regulation of CYP24. *Leuk Res,* 2006, 30: 1005-1011.

[184] Bastie JN, Balitrand N, Guillemot I, Chomienne C, Delva L. Cooperative action of 1alpha,25-dihydroxyvitamin D_3 and retinoic acid in NB4 acute promyelocytic leukemia cell differentiation is transcriptionally controlled. *Exp Cell Res,* 2005, 310: 319-330.

[185] Lou YR, Miettinen S, Kagechika H, Gronemeyer H, Tuohimaa P. Retinoic acid via RARalpha inhibits the expression of 24-hydroxylase in human prostate stromal cells. *Biochem Biophys Res Commun,* 2005, 338: 1973-1981.

[186] Sokoloski JA, Hodnick WF, Mayne ST, Cinquina C, Kim CS, Sartorelli AC. Induction of the differentiation of HL-60 promyelocytic leukemia cells by vitamin E and other antioxidants in combination with low levels of vitamin D_3: possible relationship to NF-kB. *Leukemia*, 1997, 11: 1546-1553.

[187] Kang SN, Lee MH, Kim KM, Cho D, Kim TS. Induction of human promyelocytic leukemia HL-60 cell differentiation into monocytes by silibinin: involvement of protein kinase C. *Biochem Pharmacol*, 2001, 61: 1487-1495.

[188] Danilenko M, Wang X, Studzinski GP. Carnosic acid and promotion of monocytic differentiation of HL60-G cells initiated by other agents. *J Natl Cancer Inst,* 2001, 93: 1224-1233.

[189] Danilenko M, Wang Q, Wang X, Levy J, Sharoni Y, Studzinski GP. Carnosic acid potentiates the antioxidant and prodifferentiation effects of 1alpha,25-dihydroxyvitamin D_3 in leukemia cells but does not promote elevation of basal levels of intracellular calcium. *Cancer Res*, 2003, 63: 1325-1332.

[190] Wang Q, Salman H, Danilenko M, Studzinski GP. Cooperation between antioxidants and 1,25-dihydroxyvitamin D_3 in induction of leukemia HL60 cell differentiation through the JNK/AP-1/Egr-1 pathway. *J Cell Physiol*, 2005, 204: 964-974.

[191] Kang SN, Kim SH, Chung SW, Lee MH, Kim HJ, Kim TS. Enhancement of 1 alpha,25-dihydroxyvitamin D_3-induced differentiation

of human leukaemia HL-60 cells into monocytes by parthenolide via inhibition of NF-kB activity. *Br J Pharmacol,* 2002, 135: 1235-1244.

[192] Kim SH, Kang SN, Kim HJ, Kim TS. Potentiation of 1,25-dihydroxyvitamin D_3-induced differentiation of human promyelocytic leukemia cells into monocytes by costunolide, a germacranolide sesquiterpene lactone. *Biochem Pharmacol,* 2002, 64: 1233-1242.

[193] Poon KH, Zhang J, Wang C, Tse AK, Wan CK, Fong WF. Betulinic acid enhances 1alpha,25-dihydroxyvitamin D_3-induced differentiation in human HL-60 promyelocytic leukemia cells. *Anticancer Drugs,* 2004, 15: 619-624.

[194] Ji Y, Lee HJ, Goodman C, Uskokovic M, Liby K, Sporn M, Suh N. The synthetic triterpenoid CDDO-imidazolide induces monocytic differentiation by activating the Smad and ERK signaling pathways in HL60 leukemia cells. *Mol Cancer Ther,* 2006, 5: 1452-1458.

[195] Iguchi T, Miyazawa K, Asada M, Gotoh A, Mizutani S, Ohyashiki K. Combined treatment of leukemia cells with vitamin K_2 and 1alpha,25-dihydroxy vitamin D_3 enhances monocytic differentiation along with becoming resistant to apoptosis by induction of cytoplasmic $p21^{CIP1}$. *Int J Oncol,* 2005, 27: 893-900.

[196] Amano Y, Cho Y, Matsunawa M, Komiyama K, Makishima M. Increased nuclear expression and transactivation of vitamin D receptor by the cardiotonic steroid bufalin in human myeloid leukemia cells. *J Steroid Biochem Mol Biol*, 2009, 114: 144-151.

[197] Kim SH, Yoo JC, Kim TS. Nargenicin enhances 1,25-dihydroxyvitamin D_3- and all-trans retinoic acid-induced leukemia cell differentiation via PKCbetaI/MAPK pathways. *Biochem Pharmacol,* 2009, 77: 1694-1701.

[198] Wietzke JA, Welsh J. Phytoestrogen regulation of a Vitamin D_3 receptor promoter and 1,25-dihydroxyvitamin D_3 actions in human breast cancer cells. *J Steroid Biochem Mol Biol*, 2003, 84: 149-157.

[199] Rao A, Coan A, Welsh JE, Barclay WW, Koumenis C, Cramer SD. Vitamin D receptor and p21/WAF1 are targets of genistein and 1,25-dihydroxyvitamin D_3 in human prostate cancer cells. *Cancer Res,* 2004, 64: 2143-2147.

[200] Swami S, Krishnan AV, Peehl DM, Feldman D. Genistein potentiates the growth inhibitory effects of 1,25-dihydroxyvitamin D_3 in DU145 human prostate cancer cells: role of the direct inhibition of CYP24 enzyme activity. *Mol Cell Endocrinol,* 2005, 241: 49-61.

[201] Yin Y, Ni J, Chen M, Guo Y, Yeh S. RRR-alpha-vitamin E succinate potentiates the antitumor effect of calcitriol in prostate cancer without overt side effects. *Clin Cancer Res,* 2009, 15: 190-200.

[202] Istfan NW, Person KS, Holick MF, Chen TC. 1alpha,25-Dihydroxyvitamin D and fish oil synergistically inhibit G1/S-phase transition in prostate cancer cells. *J Steroid Biochem Mol Biol*, 2007, 103: 726-730.

[203] Chiang KC, Persons KS, Istfan NW, Holick MF, Chen TC. Fish oil enhances the antiproliferative effect of 1alpha,25-dihydroxyvitamin D_3 on liver cancer cells. *Anticancer Res*, 2009, 29: 3591-3596.

[204] Sharabani H, Izumchenko E, Wang Q, Kreinin R, Steiner M, Barvish Z, Kafka M, Sharoni Y, Levy J, Uskokovic M, Studzinski GP, Danilenko M. Cooperative antitumor effects of vitamin D_3 derivatives and rosemary preparations in a mouse model of myeloid leukemia. *Int J Cancer,* 2006, 118: 3012-3021.

[205] Shabtay A, Sharabani H, Barvish Z, Kafka M, Amichay D, Levy J, Sharoni Y, Uskokovic MR, Studzinski GP, Danilenko M. Synergistic antileukemic activity of carnosic acid-rich rosemary extract and the 19-nor Gemini vitamin D analogue in a mouse model of systemic acute myeloid leukemia. *Oncology*, 2008, 75: 203-214.

[206] Miyamoto K, Kesterson RA, Yamamoto H, Taketani Y, Nishiwaki E, Tatsumi S, Inoue Y, Morita K, Takeda E, Pike JW. Structural organization of the human vitamin D receptor chromosomal gene and its promoter. *Mol Endocrinol,* 1997, 11: 1165-1179.

In: Vitamin D: Biochemistry, Nutrition ... ISBN: 978-1-61668-273-6
Editor: W. J. Stackhouse, pp. 37-66

Chapter 2

VITAMIN D RECEPTOR AGONISTS AND KIDNEY DISEASES

***Theodoros Eleftheriadis*[*1] *and Vassilios Liakopoulos*[2]**
[1]General Hospital of Serres, Serres, Greece
[2]University Hospital of Larissa, Larissa, Greece

SECTION 1: CLASSICAL ACTIONS OF VITAMIN D RECEPTOR AGONISTS AND KIDNEY DISEASES

The structure of vitamin D was described by Adolf Windaus in 1927 (1). Brunette and co workers discovered that calcitriol is synthesized in the proximal convoluted tubule of the kidney (2). Slatopolsky et al suggested the role of active vitamin D in the treatment of secondary hyperparathyroidism (SHPT) (3). A lot of progress in our understanding of the physiology of vitamin D and its role in calcium and phosphorus homeostasis has been made in the recent years.

Vitamin D is produced from 7-dehydrocholesterol in the skin by ultraviolet radiation or absorbed from dietary sources. It is then converted by the liver to 25-hydroxyvitamin D. Then it is transported to the kidneys where it is converted to 1,25-dihydroxyvitamin D, the active form of vitamin D or calcitriol. Vitamin D is not a vitamin, it is a hormone. Active vitamin D plays

* Corresponding Author: Theodoros Eleftheriadis, Department of Nephrology, General Hospital of Serres, 3rd km Serres-Drama, 62100, Serres, Greece, e-mail: teleftheriadis@yahoo.com

a central role in the regulation of calcium by increasing calcium and phosphorus absorption in the gastrointestinal tract, by stimulating osteoclast activity and stimulating calcium absorption in the distal tubule (4).

Secondary hyperparathyroidism develops in the course of chronic kidney disease and calcitriol holds a pivotal role in its pathogenesis. Progressive kidney disease is associated with a decline in production and impairment of the action of vitamin D, which leads to an inadequate serum calcium control. Calcitriol controls parathyroid cell growth and suppresses the synthesis and secretion of parathyroid hormone (PTH) by decreasing the transcription of its gene (5). Therefore, active vitamin D is a part of the therapeutic armory for the management of secondary hyperparathyroidism. Today, active vitamin D and its analogs are the mainstay of treatment to control serum PTH and most of hemodialysis patients are receiving one of these agents.

Recently, the *Klotho* gene and fibroblast growth factor (FGF)-23 have been involved in the regulation of vitamin D. *Klotho* is expressed predominantly in the distal tubule. It acts as a co-factor for the stimulation of the FGF-23 receptor permitting several cells to respond to FGF-23 (6). FGF-23 is a counter-regulatory hormone for vitamin D (7) secreted by bone cells in response to hyperphosphatemia and vitamin D administration (8). Levels of FGF-23 increase after administration of vitamin D and act on 1-a-hydroxylase reducing formation of active vitamin D. Furthermore, FGF-23 stimulates 24- and 25-hydroxylase activity enhancing the degradation of active vitamin D. (8) Calcitriol enhances the mRNA FGF-23 expression in bone cells through the binding of VDRs to the promoter region of the FGF-23 gene (9). FGF-23 knockout mice have very high calcitriol and phosphorus levels and exhibit extensive soft-tissue calcification, (10) similarly to mice carrying a *Klotho* mutation (11).

Mechanisms of Vitamin D Deficiency in Chronic Kidney Disease

In chronic kidney disease (CKD), reduced calcitriol activity, enhanced degradation of the active vitamin D and loss of VDR expression are observed contributing to the development of secondary hyperparathyroidism.

Circulating 1,25-dihydroxyvitamin D begins to decrease in stage 2 CKD. As CKD progresses its levels continue to fall following the decrease in renal mass and the reduction of 1a-hydroxylase activity.

The activity of kidney specific 1a-hydroxylase is impaired in CKD due to hyperphosphatemia, decreased filtration of the substrate 25-hydroxyvitamin D

(12) and the retention of N-terminally truncated PTH fragments or C-terminal PTH fragments (13).

The recently discovered phosphaturic hormone FGF-23 increases in the course of kidney disease as a response to hyperphosphatemia. FGF-23 can directly suppress 1-a-hydroxylase activity by decreasing 1-a-hydroxylase mRNA (14) and stimulating the 24,25-hydroxylase which leads to the degradation of 1,25-hydroxyvitamin D3 (15).

Hyperuricemia, (16) metabolic acidosis (17) and uremic toxins (18) can further suppress 1a-hydroxylase activity.

Low 25-hydroxyvitamin D levels can also lead to decreased levels of active vitamin D. Like in the general population, aging, inadequate nutritional intake, malabsorption and decreased sunlight exposure may all result in 25-hydroxyvitamin D deficiency. (19) CKD patients are often elderly, malnourished and poorly exposed to sunlight. Moreover, a decreased skin response to ultraviolet light to produce vitamin D3 from 7-dehydrocholesterol is observed in CKD. Proteinuria, especially in the nephrotic range, is another important cause of 25-hydroxy vitamin D deficiency, resulting from the loss of the 25-hydroxy vitamin D binding protein in the urine due to the impaired megalin-mediated endocytosis (20).

Severe parathyroid hyperplasia may also induce resistance to the action of vitamin D due to a decrease in VDRs in the parathyroid glands (21).

Role of Active Vitamin D in Secondary Hyperparathyroidism

1,25-dihydroxyvitamin D promotes intestinal absorption of calcium and phosphorus and bone mineralization. Vitamin D suppresses PTH levels by preventing parathyroid gland enlargement and decreasing PTH synthesis (20). Parathyroid growth is arrested in part by preventing increases in TGF-α and epidermal growth factor receptor (EGFR) (22). Parathyroid hyperplasia correlates with enhanced co-expression of TGF-α and its receptor (epidermal growth factor receptor) (23). Active vitamin D suppresses PTH synthesis and parathyroid cell proliferation through a genomic activity. This genomic effect is regulated by the vitamin D receptors (VDR). VDR forms a heterodimer with the retinoid X receptor that enables the complex active vitamin D and VDR to bind with high affinity to the vitamin D response element on the transcription promoters of vitamin D sensitive genes (8). Furthermore, a rapid non-genomic effect of active vitamin D has been detected in intestinal cells (24).

The activation of VDR suppresses PTH secretion also by enhancing the sensitivity of the parathyroid glands to calcium. This is accomplished by an increase in serum calcium and subsequent activation of the calcium sensing receptor (CaSR) and by direct action on the number of CaSRs in the parathyroid glands (25).

Besides the parathyroid glands, vitamin D receptors have been detected in a number of tissues with probably different roles. In the intestine they promote calcium and phosphorus absorption, in the kidney they promote calcium reabsorption and regulate vitamin D, in the bone they regulate bone formation and reabsorption, in the pancreas they regulate insulin secretion, in the cardiovascular system they have inhibitory actions on rennin and antiproliferative effects and in the immune system they posses immunomodulatory properties (8).

Calcific uremic arteriolopathy (previously calciphylaxis) is an uncommon and life threatening complication occurring in patients with End Stage Renal Disease (ESRD). It has been associated with the use of Vitamin D (26). However, this has not been proven in non-uremia associated calciphylaxis (27) and beneficial effects of vitamin D analogs with less calcemic and phosphatemic actions (like paricalcitol) have been documented even in dialysis patients (28).

The 2003 K/DOQI guidelines for bone metabolism and disease in CKD recommend that active vitamin D should be administered if intact PTH levels are greater then 300 pmol/L. Treatment with vitamin D should be withheld if serum calcium is greater than 9.5 mg/dL or serum phosphorus persistently greater then 4.6 mg/dL (29).

However, there are some data regarding more aggressive use of vitamin D in CKD patients that put these recommendations into question.

A small randomized placebo controlled study showed improved bone health as assessed by dual-energy X-ray absorptiometry, bone density tests and serum bone biomarkers in predialysis CKD patients receiving alfacalcidol (30). In a similar population early administration of alfacalcidol resulted in significant improvement in bone morphology and biochemical indices compared with the placebo group (31). Paricalcitol has shown to improve bone morphology and indices in experimental or small studies when compared to calcitriol (32, 33). Based on these findings and on the identification that bone cell VDR activation is prerequisite for the maintenance of normal bone formation (34) some authors consider active vitamin D treatment in CKD regardless of bone turnover status (35). However, the most interesting and important data are these regarding the effect of vitamin D treatment on patient survival.

25-Hydroxyvitamin D in Chronic Kidney Disease

The 2003 K/DOQI guidelines for bone metabolism and disease in CKD recommend that if the serum level of 25-hydroxyvitamin D is <30 ng/mL, supplementation with vitamin D2, (ergocalciferol) should be initiated (29).

25-hydroxy vitamin D deficiency is a common finding in patients with CKD especially in those with severe proteinuria. Secondary hyperparathyroidism develops almost in all patients with 25-hydroxy vitamin D deficiency (36). In contrast to the general population there is a positive relationship between 25-hydroxy vitamin D levels and 1,25-dihydroxy vitamin D levels in CKD.

A number of studies have addressed the effects of 25-hydroxyvitamin D administration on secondary hyperparathyroidism in CKD. Zisman et al, showed that therapy with ergocalciferol in CKD stage 3 and 4 could result in a rise of 25-hydroxyvitamin D slightly above the 30 ng/mL threshold and a small decrease in PTH mainly in patients with stage 3 CKD (37). Chandra et al in a randomized controlled trial in a similar population observed a 50 ng/mL mean value for 25-hydroxyvitamin D and a substantial decrease in PTH values for the treatment group. However, a high variability in PTH values was observed resulting in a non statistically significant difference (38). Al-Aly et al showed that only 50% of the patients receiving 25-hydroxyvitamin D treatment successfully raised its levels and these were the ones with a significant decrease in PTH (39).

Administration of 25-hydroxyvitamin D has been shown to correct its levels in the dialysis population with beneficial effects on relevant biochemical markers (40, 41). As already mentioned an association between 25-hydroxyvitamin D levels and survival has been described in CKD patients as well as in the general population. From the above findings its use in deficient patients is justified.

Vitamin D and the Calcium Sensing Receptor

Calcimimetics (Cinacalcet is currently the approved agent for the treatment of SHPT in dialysis patients) are non calcium agents that bind to the calcium sensing receptor (CaSR) which is expressed on parathyroid chief cells, increase cell sensitivity to extracellular calcium and suppress PTH secretion independently of vitamin D. Calcium is still needed in order to activate the CaSR and control PTH secretion. Concerns have been raised about the use of cinacalcet and the potential for hypocalcemia, increased calciuria and hyperphosphatemia. The use of vitamin D is required in over 75% of patients receiving cinacalcet and there have been questions about the possible role of cinacalcet in worsening calcitriol deficiency through direct or indirect inhibitory effects on 1-a-hydroxylase (42).

The combined use of cinacalcet and active vitamin D compounds has been proposed based on the experimental findings that active vitamin D increases the sensitivity of the CaSR (43) and plays an important role in its regulation (25).

The addition of cinacalcet treatment on top of optimal standard therapy with active vitamin D resulted in better control of SHPT (44, 45) and in a higher proportion of dialysis patients achieving the K/DOQI treatment goals for calcium, phosphorus and PTH (46). In the OPTIMA study patients receiving the combination of cinacalcet and vitamin D derivatives had better results regarding their previously poorly controlled SHPT. The use of Cinacalcet allowed a reduction in the dose of vitamin D by one fifth (47). In another study the combination of cinacalcet with low dose active vitamin D resulted in an improved control of mineral metabolism and a high proportion of patients achieving the K/DOQI treatment goals (48).

Forms of Vitamin D

Native vitamin D (Ergocalciferol – vitamin D2 and Cholecalciferol-vitamin D3): Their use has been recommended in 25-hydroxyvitamin D deficient CKD patients. No difference between the two has been described with regard to the degree of response of 25-hydroxyvitamin D levels (12).

Active vitamin D Calcitriol (1,25-dihydroxyvitamin D3): It is the most well-studied form of vitamin D with very good results regarding control of SHPT and patient survival.

In an effort to decrease the toxicity of vitamin D therapy a number of vitamin D analogs have been introduced. They are considered to have lesser calcemic and phosphatemic effects but retain the ability to suppress PTH. Currently 3 vitamin D analogs and two synthetic prohormones are used in the treatment of secondary hyperparathyroidism.

Paricalcitol (19-nor-1,25-dihydroxyvitamin D2) has been shown effective in suppressing PTH with lesser concomitant increases in calcium and phosphate levels. In contrast to calcitriol, paricalcitol is more selective to the parathyroid gland and does not upregulate the VDR receptor in the intestine (49). It also stimulates intestinal calcium transport proteins (e.g. calbindin) in a lesser degree than calcitriol (50). However, hypercalcemia can still be encountered especially if PTH is suppressed to low levels. (51) Finally, an advantage of paricalcitol vs. calcitriol in terms of hospitalization rates and survival has been shown in recent studies (52-54). It is available for both oral and intravenous use.

Maxacalcitol (22-oxacalcitriol) is a structurally modified vitamin D3 where the insertion of an oxygen in the 22 position results in decreased binding affinity for both the VDR and vitamin D binding protein, leading in a rapid clearance from the circulation. This analog, which is in use in Asia, effectively suppresses PTH, with a safer profile and possibly ameliorates the effects of PTH on bone (5). It is available orally.

Falecalcitriol is a vitamin D3 analog where hydrogen has been substituted with fluorine in the 26 and 27 positions. It has a prolonged biological activity due to its decreased metabolism and has been effective in PTH suppression (5).

Two prohormones, *1-a-hydroxyvitamin D3 (alfa-calcidol)* and *1-a-hydroxyvitamin D2 (doxercalciferol)* are also in clinical use. Alfacalcidol becomes 25-hydroxylated in the liver and has been shown to have similar activity to calcitriol. Doxercalciferol becomes also 25-hydroxylate in the liver and seemingly has lesser toxicity (21). Both prohormones are available for oral and intravenous use.

Vitamin D and Survival

Administration of active vitamin D to dialysis patients seems to be associated with a survival advantage. This is supported by a number of studies.

A study by Marco et al showed that the *Bsm*I polymorphism of the VDR influences survival in hemodialysis patients. This could be attributed to either a direct modification of the sensitivity or expression of the VDR in target cells or to induced differences in 1,25 dihydroxyvitamin D3 levels (55). The same study suggested that patients receiving calcitriol treatment had a survival advantage over untreated patients.

The use of injectable active forms of active vitamin D has been linked with a survival advantage in hemodialysis patients in a number of studies. Both calcitriol and paricalcitol have been shown to reduce mortality in this population (56-58).

Paricalcitol, as well as, 1-a-hydroxyvitamin D2 have been associated with improved survival advantage over calcitriol. Paricalcitol also reduced admission rates compared with calcitriol (52-54).

Oral forms of active vitamin D have been also reported to have a positive impact on survival in hemodialysis population (59). Similar results have been reported for low dose 1-a hydroxyvitamin D3 and cardiovascular mortality in a group of 242 hemodialysis patients (60).

In predialysis patients with chronic kidney disease similar results have been reported. Oral calcitriol treatment has been associated with improved survival in a cohort of 520 US patients with CKD stage 3-5 (61). In another study involving 1418 patients with hyperparathyroidism and CKD stage 3-4 oral calcitriol was also associated with lower mortality (62).

Furthermore, in a retrospective study by Wolf et al in a cohort of 825 incident hemodialysis patients, a correlation of early (90 days) mortality and low levels of 25-hydroxyvitamin D was shown. In the same study, treatment with active vitamin D was associated with improved survival (57). Similarly, in the general population, low 25-hydroxyvitamin D levels were independently associated with all cause mortality (63).

Interestingly a large historical cohort study showed that while elevated serum calcium, phosphorus and PTH were independently associated with increased mortality, the vitamin D–associated survival benefit persisted within each metabolite quintile (58). Thus factors beyond the effects of vitamin D on bone metabolism likely contribute to the survival advantage of VDR agonist administration (64).

Section 2: Non-Classical Actions of Vitamin D Receptor Agonists and Kidney Diseases

From an evolutionary point of view, the fact that vitamin D has appeared more than 500 million years ago in lower non-vertebrate life forms, which did not have a skeleton and used to live in the rich in calcium oceans , makes the acquisition of other roles quite possible (65). Furthermore, the possible pleiotropic roles of vitamin D can be supported by the presence of its receptor, the vitamin D receptor (VDR) in a wide variety of tissues (65, 66).

Although there is discrepancy about the additional benefits of less calcemic vitamin D analogs administration in the survival of patients with end stage renal disease (ESRD), large retrospective studies agree that both calcitriol and its analogs paricalcitol or doxercalciferol increase survival in this group of patients (52, 53, 58). This benefit could be the result of an anti-inflammatory/immunomodulatory effect of VDR agonists. ESRD patients are under a state of chronic inflammation. Uremia per se, rupture of skin continuity during AV access puncture, central venous catheters, contact of blood with dialysis membranes, endotoxins in dialysis solution and certainly the various co-morbid conditions, all lead to monocyte pre-activation and production of pro-inflammatory cytokines, such as interleukin (IL)-1, IL-6, IL-12 and tumor necrosis factor (TNF)-α, resulting in a subclinical systemic inflammation (67). This systemic inflammation contributes to the mortality of hemodialysis (HD) patients, since it has been incriminated for atherosclerosis progression (68, 69), malnutrition (70), inadequate immune response to infections and vaccines (71-77), and resistance to recombinant human erythropoietin (78, 79).

In addition, there are indications that VDR agonists may also play a beneficial role in patients with chronic renal failure (CRF) before the initiation of dialysis. A prospective study confirmed that low serum level of $25(OH)D_3$, which is the precursor of the active VDR agonist $1,25(OH)_2D_3$ or calcitriol, is a negative prognostic factor for both progression to ESRD and death (80). Another prospective study showed that paricalcitol administration in patients with CRF reduced proteinuria, even in those patients that were treated with blockers of the renin-angiotensin system (RAS), i.e. angiotensin converting enzyme inhibitors (ACEIs) or angiotensin II type I receptor blockers (ARBs) (81). Non-traditional mechanisms of action related to the local renal response to injury and discussed below may be responsible for these observations.

The Immunomodulatory Action of VDR Agonists and the Kidney Diseases

Vitamin D receptor is expressed in antigen presenting cells (APCs) and stimulated T-cells and B-cells (82-85). The same cells also express the enzyme 1α-hydroxylase, which converts the $25(OH)D_3$ to the active $1,25(OH)_2D_3$. Various mediators of inflammation have been shown to increase 1α-hydroxylase expression. In the case of inflammation, very high concentrations of calcitriol can be achieved locally because 1α-hydroxylase in macrophages is not regulated through the known negative feedback loops from the renal tubules (86-89). In addition, interferon (IFN)-γ inhibits calcitriol catabolism because it decreases 24-hydroxylase expression (90, 91).

Animal studies showed that $1,25(OH)_2D_3$ and its analogs prevent various autoimmune diseases (92-100). Additionally, $1,25(OH)_2D_3$ and its analogs prolong survival of various organ allografts in animals (101-104). A synergism between VDR agonists and classical immunosuppressive agents, such as cyclosporine, FK-506, rapamycin and mycophenolate mofetil, was confirmed (103, 105-109). This synergism could be the result of the VDR agonists' action on APCs, since classical immunosuppressive agents act mainly at the level of the T-cell. Interestingly, despite allograft survival prolongation, VDR agonists do not compromise resistance to opportunistic infections (110). The increased vitamin D mediated expression of antimicrobial peptides, such as cathelicidin, could contribute to the last observation (89, 111-113).

Clinical observations also showed that in many chronic inflammatory autoimmune diseases like inflammatory bowel disease (114, 115), multiple sclerosis (116-118), systemic lupus erythematosus (119), diabetes mellitus type I (120, 121) and rheumatoid arthritis (122-124), serum levels of vitamin D are low and in many cases its administration has beneficial effects. In the general population low serum $25(OH)D_3$ levels have been correlated with increased CRP, increased incidence of tuberculosis and decreased skin delayed hypersensitivity reaction (125-127).

It is now known that VDR agonists modulate almost any step of the adaptive immune response. At the level of the antigen presenting cell (APC), vitamin D decreases the expression of major histocompatibility class II (MHCII) and of the co-stimulatory molecules CD80, CD86 and CD40 (128, 129). Additionally, VDR agonists promote a shifting from Th1 phenotype to Th2 phenotype and therefore indirectly inhibit cytotoxic CD8+ T-lymphocytes and APCs function (130-132). Furthermore, VDR agonists induce regulatory T-cell production (129, 133), while they decrease the differentiation of Th0 cells to T helper lymphocytes type 17 (Th17) cells, which play a significant role in inflammation and autoimmune diseases (133). Regarding humoral immunity, VDR agonists inhibit B-cell differentiation to plasma cells and thus antibody production (134, 135). Vitamin D also inhibits the production of the pro-inflammatory cytokines IL-1 and TNF-α by monocytes and macrophages attenuating the inflammatory response (136, 137). Interestingly, the chemotactic, phagocytic and bacteriocidal activity of monocytes and macrophages are increased by vitamin D (113).

In HD patients $1\alpha(OH)D_3$ partially restores IL-2 production by peripheral blood mononuclear cells (PBMCs) in culture (138). Furtehrmore, $1,25(OH)_2D_3$ increases IL-2 production and decreases TNF-α production by stimulated HD patients-derived PBMCs (139). In another study, $1,25(OH)_2D_3$ failed to restore the proliferation of stimulated PBMCs from HD patients, but enhanced proliferation was observed selectively in PBMCs derived from HD patients with low serum $1,25(OH)_2D_3$ (140). Additionally, $1,25(OH)_2D_3$ administration reduces IL-1 and IL-6 levels in the serum of HD patients (141).

Paricalcitol has anti-inflammatory properties as well. In healthy volunteers it inhibits basal and lipopolysaccharide (LPS)-induced production of the chemokine IL-8, which plays important role in acute inflammation, and of the pro-inflammatory cytokine TNF-α by the PBMCs (142). Interestingly, in the presence of LPS, and in contrary to calcitriol, paricalcitol does not inhibit osteoprotegerin (OPG) production by PBMCs (143). Considering that about 65% of OPG is produced by B-cells with the help of T-cells (144), it is possible that compared to calcitriol, paricalcitol exerts its anti-inflammatory effect with less osteolytic activity. In a pilot study in predialysis patients, oral paricalcitol reduced proteinuria and inflammation as assessed by serum CRP (145).

Experimentally, the anti-inflammatory effect of VDR agonists at the level of the kidney has also been verified (146). In a mouse model of unilateral ureteral obstruction, monocytes and T-cells infiltrate the interstitium of the obstructed kidney and produce TNF-α. TNF-α through the transcription factor NF-κB induces the production of the chemokine RANTES by renal tubular cells, which promotes further kidney infiltration by monocytes and T-cells closing a vicious circle that preserves the inflammatory reaction and promotes the kidney destruction. Paricalcitol administration breaks the above vicious circle and attenuates inflammation, since it augments VDR expression in renal tubular cells. Then the activated by paricalcitol VDR sequesters the NF-κB and prevents the transcription of RANTES.

Low $25(OH)D_3$ is a common finding, especially in the context of kidney disease (80, 147). Theoretically, the restoration of $25(OH)D_3$ levels could have more impressive immunomodulatory/anti-inflammatory effects than the administration of active VDR agonists (the doses of which are restricted by the possibility of hypercalcemia) in patients with CRF. The reason is the high capacity of macrophages to convert $25(OH)D_3$ to active calcitriol locally at the site of inflammation (87-91). This is in accordance with a study in patients with CRF, which showed that low serum levels of $25(OH)D_3$ and not of $1,25(OH)_2D_3$ was a negative prognostic factor for both progression to ESRD and death (80). In the general population serum $25(OH)D_3$ levels below 20ng/ml are considered as vitamin D deficiency and less than 30ng/ml as vitamin D insufficiency. But these lower limits arose from studies that evaluated the effect of vitamin D on parathyroid hormone level and bone metabolism (148, 149). Similarly, the K/DOQI clinical practice guidelines for bone metabolism and disease in chronic kidney diseases suggests ergocalciferol supplementation when serum $25(OH)D_3$ levels are below 30ng/ml. This guideline is opinion based and only parameters of bone metabolism are considered (29). The optimal serum $25(OH)D_3$ level for the function of the immune system is not defined yet for both the general population and for the patients with CRF, with the particular features of vitamin D metabolism.

Despite the fact that the immunomodulatory/anti-inflammatory properties of VDR agonists have been confirmed, we cannot expect miracles. In VDR knockout mice there are some relatively slight in vitro, and after antigenic stimulation, in vivo disturbances of helper T-cells function but not a dramatic immune system dysfunction, such as spontaneous autoimmune diseases (93). The picture in patients with hereditary vitamin D dependent rickets type II and point VDR mutations is similar (150). Therefore it is quite possible that VDR agonists will not replace classical immunosuppressive agents. On the other hand, the lack of a very potent immunomodulatory effect could be useful in the subclinical systemic inflammation of CRF and HD. Certainly the synergism between the VDR agonists and the classical immunosuppressive agents is also promising, and deserves clinical evaluation.

VDR Agonists, Fibrosis and Kidney Diseases

Inflammation is the universal initial response of the organism to any injurious agent. In case of injurious agent persistence, chronic inflammation and tissue repair coexist. In mammals, tissue/organ regeneration is restricted and the repair process involves fibrosis. Excessive fibrosis leads to organ failure (151, 152). Actually, inflammation and fibrosis are indispensable components of the same process, i.e. of the body's response to injury.

Tissue repair is a highly complex process that includes epithelial cell proliferation, angiogenesis, and extracellular matrix (ECM) production (153). The last is responsible for fibrosis and the major players are the myofibroblats, which produce ECM (154, 155), and the cytokine transforming growth factor (TGF)-β1 (156). Although TGF-β1 is produced by almost any cell type, its major source is the macrophages that infiltrate the site of injury.

TGF-β1 is produced in a latent form and stored within the ECM (157). Various factors, such as inflammation, mechanical stress, angiotensin II, high glucose and endothelin-1 by means of acidic pH, expression of $\alpha_v\beta_6$ integrins or matrix metalloproteinases (MMPs) and activation of thrombospondin-1 or plasmin activate latent TGF-β1. Activated TGF-β1 binds its type II receptor, which is then connected to type I receptor, leading to recruitment and phosphorylation of the cytoplasmic SMAD2 or 3 (158, 159). Phosphorylated SMAD2/3 form complexes with SMAD4 that enter into the nucleus and start the transcription of various genes including those that are required for myofibroblast formation, components of the ECM, connective tissue growth factor, which is a mediator of some TGF-β1 actions (160), SMAD7, which by facilitating TGF-β1 receptor type I and SMAD2/3 degradation acts as a negative feedback loop in the above signal transduction pathway (161), and others. MMPs production is decreased, and thus ECM degradation is inhibited. Interestingly, TGF-β1 transcription is increased, forming a positive feedback loop that could preserve ECM production and fibrosis. Recent studies revealed that apart from the above classical TGF-β1 signal transduction pathway, many others also exist (162). There are also a number of other factors that may interfere with the above signal transduction pathway. Angiotensin II and advanced glycation end products (AGEs), through the extracellular signal-regulated kinase (ERK)/p38 kinase pathway, can directly phosphorylate the SMAD2/3 and initiate the vicious cycle of fibrosis (163-165).

Although experimental studies confirm the beneficial effect of VDR agonists in various types of glomerulopathies (166-169), renal interstitial fibrosis will be mainly analyzed further because this pattern of renal fibrosis is a common feature of most kidney diseases and is well correlated with the progression of renal damage (170, 171). Renal injury leads to inflammation and infiltration of the interstitium with macrophages. Macrophages produce TGF-β1, which promotes myofibroblast formation. In the kidney interstitium, about 50% of the myofibroblasts are derived from local fibroblasts, 35% from epithelial renal tubular cells to mesenchymal cells transition and 15% from bone marrow derived fibrocytes and mesenchymal cells (151, 172-175). Interestingly, TGF-β1 induces its own production by myofibroblasts and also is a potent chemo-attractant for the macrophages, forming a positive feedback loop that preserves the fibrotic process (176).

In vitro and in vivo experimental models confirmed that VDR agonists interfering with TGF-β1 signal transduction attenuate renal interstitial fibrosis and preserve renal function. VDR agonists decrease TGF-β1 production and its type I receptor expression (177). They also inhibit TGF-β1 signal transduction by decreasing SMAD3 expression or through a direct interaction of the VDR with the SMAD3 (178, 179). VDR agonists suppress connective tissue TGF, which is a mediator of some TGF-β1 functions (180). In a model of unilateral ureteral obstruction VDR agonists prevent epithelial to mesenchymal transition through the inhibition of the transcription factor Snail, which is a product of the classical TGF-β1 signal transduction pathway (177). Interestingly, in a model of subtotal nephrectomy, VDR agonists showed synergism with enalapril and attenuated renal inflammation and fibrosis (181). Macrophage infiltration was decreased due to reduced MCP-1 expression and TGF-β1 expression was also decreased due to inhibition of SMAD2 phosphorylation.

The interaction of VDR agonists with RAS is also very important, since all the components of the RAS axis promote renal fibrosis (163-165). In vitro and in vivo experimental models showed that VDR agonists, independently of serum calcium level (182), prevent transcription factors binding to the cAMP response element of the renin promoter reducing its systemic and local renal levels (182-185). Additionally, by inhibiting the vascular endothelial growth factor (VEGF) expression through the angiotensinII/p38 kinase pathway, VDR agonists exert a beneficial effect on the glomerulus, as well (183). Diabetes mellitus induction in VDR knockout mice is accompanied by increased local renal expression of renin, angiotensin II and angiotensin II receptor, increased ECM production and worse renal prognosis compared to wild type counterparts (186). The synergism between VDR agonists and ACEIs or ARBs is also very interesting and clinically significant. In a model of diabetic nephropathy, paricalcitol exerts synergism with losartan in decreasing the production of TGF-β1, MCP-1 and fibronectin (187). Besides the interstitium, the benefits of the above synergism are extended to the glomerulus, with a better restoration of the slit diaphragm structural proteins and decreased proteinuria compared to the administration of each compound separately. The beneficial effects of VDR agonists' co-administration with RAS blockers were attributed to the intrarenal renin and angiotensin II blockage by the VDR agonists observed in this study. However, RAS independent pathways should also play an important role.

SUMMARY

In-depth research in the past two decades has revealed many of the potential mechanisms in which vitamin D is involved in the initiation and maintenance of calcium and phosphorus disturbances in CKD. Vitamin D holds a pivotal role in the treatment of secondary hyperparathyroidism and bone disease that are associated with CKD. Early parathyroid gland VDR activation is likely to be the best way to prevent the development of irreversible nodular hyperplasia, which is the major contributor to resistant hyperparathyroidism in ESRD.

Clinical studies confirmed that vitamin D receptor (VDR) agonist administration offers a survival benefit in hemodialysis patients and may help in preservation of renal function in predialysis patients. Accumulated clinical and mainly experimental data support that in the context of kidney disease VDR agonists exert their beneficial effect not only due to their action on calcium and phosphorus homeostasis, but also through modulation of the response to injury. They attenuate systemic and renal inflammation and they affect tissue repair process reducing renal fibrosis.

Further clinical research is needed to answer questions including issues like the optimal time to screen for vitamin D deficiency, the effects of treatment of vitamin D deficiency, potential differences between different forms of vitamin D and to define the optimal dosage, duration, goals, and outcomes of treatment with vitamin D.

REFERENCES

[1] Wolf G. The discovery of vitamin D: the contribution of Adolf Windaus. *J Nutr* 2004; 134: 1299-1302.

[2] Brunette MG, Chan M, Ferriere C, Roberts KD. Site of 1,25(OH)2 vitamin D3 synthesis in the kidney. *Nature* 1978; 276: 287-289.

[3] Slatopolsky E, Weerts C, Thielan J, Horst R, *et al.* Marked suppression of secondary hyperparathyroidism by intravenous administration of 1,25-dihydroxy-cholecalciferol in uremic patients. *J Clin Invest* 1984; 74: 2136-2143.

[4] Bhan I, Thadhani R. Vitamin D therapy for chronic kidney disease. *Semin Nephrol* 2009; 29: 85-93.

[5] Martin KJ, Gonzalez EA. Vitamin D analogs: actions and role in the treatment of secondary hyperparathyroidism. *Semin Nephrol* 2004; 24: 456-459.

[6] Patel TV, Singh AK. Role of vitamin D in chronic kidney disease. *Semin Nephrol* 2009; 29: 113-121.

[7] Liu S, Tang W, Zhou J, Stubbs JR, *et al.* Fibroblast growth factor 23 is a counter-regulatory phosphaturic hormone for vitamin D. *J Am Soc Nephrol* 2006; 17: 1305-1315.

[8] Cozzolino M, Ciceri P, Volpi EM, Olivi L, *et al.* Pathophysiology of calcium and phosphate metabolism impairment in chronic kidney disease. *Blood Purif* 2009; 27: 338-344.

[9] Kruse K, Woelfel D, Strom TM. Loss of renal phosphate wasting in a child with autosomal dominant hypophosphatemic rickets caused by a FGF23 mutation. *Horm Res* 2001; 55: 305-308.

[10] Sitara D, Razzaque MS, Hesse M, Yoganathan S, *et al.* Homozygous ablation of fibroblast growth factor-23 results in hyperphosphatemia and impaired skeletogenesis, and reverses hypophosphatemia in Phex-deficient mice. *Matrix Biol* 2004; 23: 421-432.

[11] Kuro-o M, Matsumura Y, Aizawa H, Kawaguchi H, *et al.* Mutation of the mouse klotho gene leads to a syndrome resembling ageing. *Nature* 1997; 390: 45-51.

[12] Al-Badr W, Martin KJ. Vitamin D and kidney disease. *Clin J Am Soc Nephrol* 2008; 3: 1555-1560.

[13] Usatii M, Rousseau L, Demers C, Petit JL, *et al.* Parathyroid hormone fragments inhibit active hormone and hypocalcemia-induced 1,25(OH)2D synthesis. *Kidney Int* 2007; 72: 1330-1335.

[14] Perwad F, Zhang MY, Tenenhouse HS, Portale AA. Fibroblast growth factor 23 impairs phosphorus and vitamin D metabolism in vivo and suppresses 25-hydroxyvitamin D-1alpha-hydroxylase expression in vitro. *Am J Physiol Renal Physiol* 2007; 293: F1577-1583.

[15] Williams ME. Chronic kidney disease/bone and mineral metabolism: the imperfect storm. *Semin Nephrol* 2009; 29: 97-104.

[16] Vanholder R, Patel S, Hsu CH. Effect of uric acid on plasma levels of 1,25(OH)2D in renal failure. *J Am Soc Nephrol* 1993; 4: 1035-1038.

[17] Lu KC, Lin SH, Yu FC, Chyr SH, *et al.* Influence of metabolic acidosis on serum 1,25(OH)2D3 levels in chronic renal failure. *Miner Electrolyte Metab* 1995; 21: 398-402.

[18] Hsu CH, Vanholder R, Patel S, De Smet RR, *et al.* Subfractions in uremic plasma ultrafiltrate inhibit calcitriol metabolism. *Kidney Int* 1991; 40: 868-873.

[19] Holick MF. Vitamin D: importance in the prevention of cancers, type 1 diabetes, heart disease, and osteoporosis. *Am J Clin Nutr* 2004; 79: 362-371.

[20] Andress DL. Vitamin D treatment in chronic kidney disease. *Semin Dial* 2005; 18: 315-321.

[21] Bover J, Andres E, Lloret MJ, Aguilar A, *et al.* Dietary and pharmacological control of calcium and phosphate metabolism in dialysis patients. *Blood Purif* 2009; 27: 369-386.

[22] Cozzolino M, Lu Y, Finch J, Slatopolsky E, *et al.* p21WAF1 and TGF-alpha mediate parathyroid growth arrest by vitamin D and high calcium. *Kidney Int* 2001; 60: 2109-2117.

[23] Arcidiacono MV, Sato T, Alvarez-Hernandez D, Yang J, *et al.* EGFR activation increases parathyroid hyperplasia and calcitriol resistance in kidney disease. *J Am Soc Nephrol* 2008; 19: 310-320.

[24] Portale AA, Halloran BP, Morris RC, Jr. Physiologic regulation of the serum concentration of 1,25-dihydroxyvitamin D by phosphorus in normal men. *J Clin Invest* 1989; 83: 1494-1499.

[25] Brown AJ, Zhong M, Finch J, Ritter C, *et al.* Rat calcium-sensing receptor is regulated by vitamin D but not by calcium. *Am J Physiol* 1996; 270: F454-460.

[26] Fine A, Zacharias J. Calciphylaxis is usually non-ulcerating: risk factors, outcome and therapy. *Kidney Int* 2002; 61: 2210-2217.

[27] Nigwekar SU, Wolf M, Sterns RH, Hix JK. Calciphylaxis from nonuremic causes: a systematic review. *Clin J Am Soc Nephrol* 2008; 3: 1139-1143.

[28] Vargemezis V, Liakopoulos V, Kriki P, Panagoutsos S, *et al.* Pivotal Role of Paricalcitol in the Treatment of Calcific Uremic Arteriolopathy in the Presence of a Parathyroid Adenoma. *Am J Kidney Dis* 2010; 55(1): 144-147

[29] K/DOQI clinical practice guidelines for bone metabolism and disease in chronic kidney disease. *Am J Kidney Dis* 2003; 42: S1-201.

[30] Rix M, Eskildsen P, Olgaard K. Effect of 18 months of treatment with alfacalcidol on bone in patients with mild to moderate chronic renal failure. *Nephrol Dial Transplant* 2004; 19: 870-876.

[31] Hamdy NA, Kanis JA, Beneton MN, Brown CB, *et al.* Effect of alfacalcidol on natural course of renal bone disease in mild to moderate renal failure. *BMJ* 1995; 310: 358-363.

[32] Balint E, Marshall CF, Sprague SM. Effect of the vitamin D analogues paricalcitol and calcitriol on bone mineral in vitro. *Am J Kidney Dis* 2000; 36: 789-796.

[33] Monier-Faugere MC, Mawad H, Malluche HH. Opposite effects of calcitriol and paricalcitol on the parathyroid hormone-(1-84)/large carboxy-terminal-parathyroid hormone fragments ratio in patients with stage 5 chronic kidney disease. *Clin J Am Soc Nephrol* 2007; 2: 1255-1260.

[34] Panda DK, Miao D, Bolivar I, Li J, *et al.* Inactivation of the 25-hydroxyvitamin D 1alpha-hydroxylase and vitamin D receptor demonstrates independent and interdependent effects of calcium and vitamin D on skeletal and mineral homeostasis. *J Biol Chem* 2004; 279: 16754-16766.

[35] Andress DL. Adynamic bone in patients with chronic kidney disease. *Kidney Int* 2008; 73: 1345-1354.

[36] Gonzalez EA, Sachdeva A, Oliver DA, Martin KJ. Vitamin D insufficiency and deficiency in chronic kidney disease. A single center observational study. *Am J Nephrol* 2004; 24: 503-510.

[37] Zisman AL, Hristova M, Ho LT, Sprague SM. Impact of ergocalciferol treatment of vitamin D deficiency on serum parathyroid hormone concentrations in chronic kidney disease. *Am J Nephrol* 2007; 27: 36-43.

[38] Chandra P, Binongo JN, Ziegler TR, Schlanger LE, *et al.* Cholecalciferol (vitamin D3) therapy and vitamin D insufficiency in patients with chronic kidney disease: a randomized controlled pilot study. *Endocr Pract* 2008; 14: 10-17.

[39] Al-Aly Z, Qazi RA, Gonzalez EA, Zeringue A, *et al.* Changes in serum 25-hydroxyvitamin D and plasma intact PTH levels following treatment with ergocalciferol in patients with CKD. *Am J Kidney Dis* 2007; 50: 59-68.

[40] Jean G, Terrat JC, Vanel T, Hurot JM, *et al.* Daily oral 25-hydroxycholecalciferol supplementation for vitamin D deficiency in haemodialysis patients: effects on mineral metabolism and bone markers. *Nephrol Dial Transplant* 2008; 23: 3670-3676.

[41] Blair D, Byham-Gray L, Lewis E, McCaffrey S. Prevalence of vitamin D [25(OH)D] deficiency and effects of supplementation with

ergocalciferol (vitamin D2) in stage 5 chronic kidney disease patients. *J Ren Nutr* 2008; 18: 375-382.

[42] Drueke TB, Ritz E. Treatment of secondary hyperparathyroidism in CKD patients with cinacalcet and/or vitamin D derivatives. *Clin J Am Soc Nephrol* 2009; 4: 234-241.

[43] Delmez JA, Tindira C, Grooms P, Dusso A, *et al.* Parathyroid hormone suppression by intravenous 1,25-dihydroxyvitamin D. A role for increased sensitivity to calcium. *J Clin Invest* 1989; 83: 1349-1355.

[44] Block GA, Martin KJ, de Francisco AL, Turner SA, *et al.* Cinacalcet for secondary hyperparathyroidism in patients receiving hemodialysis. *N Engl J Med* 2004; 350: 1516-1525.

[45] indberg JS, Culleton B, Wong G, Borah MF, *et al.* Cinacalcet HCl, an oral calcimimetic agent for the treatment of secondary hyperparathyroidism in hemodialysis and peritoneal dialysis: a randomized, double-blind, multicenter study. *J Am Soc Nephrol* 2005; 16: 800-807.

[46] Moe SM, Chertow GM, Coburn JW, Quarles LD, *et al.* Achieving NKF-K/DOQI bone metabolism and disease treatment goals with cinacalcet HCl. *Kidney Int* 2005; 67: 760-771.

[47] Messa P, Macario F, Yaqoob M, Bouman K, *et al.* The OPTIMA study: assessing a new cinacalcet (Sensipar/Mimpara) treatment algorithm for secondary hyperparathyroidism. *Clin J Am Soc Nephrol* 2008; 3: 36-45.

[48] Chertow GM, Blumenthal S, Turner S, Roppolo M, *et al.* Cinacalcet hydrochloride (Sensipar) in hemodialysis patients on active vitamin D derivatives with controlled PTH and elevated calcium x phosphate. *Clin J Am Soc Nephrol* 2006; 1: 305-312.

[49] Takahashi F, Finch JL, Denda M, Dusso AS, *et al.* A new analog of 1,25-(OH)2D3, 19-NOR-1,25-(OH)2D2, suppresses serum PTH and parathyroid gland growth in uremic rats without elevation of intestinal vitamin D receptor content. *Am J Kidney Dis* 1997; 30: 105-112.

[50] Brown AJ, Finch J, Slatopolsky E. Differential effects of 19-nor-1,25-dihydroxyvitamin D(2) and 1,25-dihydroxyvitamin D(3) on intestinal calcium and phosphate transport. *J Lab Clin Med* 2002; 139: 279-284.

[51] Martin KJ, Gonzalez EA, Gellens ME, Hamm LL, *et al.* Therapy of secondary hyperparathyroidism with 19-nor-1alpha,25-dihydroxyvitamin D2. *Am J Kidney Dis* 1998; 32: S61-66.

[52] Teng M, Wolf M, Lowrie E, Ofsthun N, *et al.* Survival of patients undergoing hemodialysis with paricalcitol or calcitriol therapy. *N Engl J Med* 2003; 349: 446-456.

[53] Tentori F, Hunt WC, Stidley CA, Rohrscheib MR, *et al.* Mortality risk among hemodialysis patients receiving different vitamin D analogs. *Kidney Int* 2006; 70: 1858-1865.

[54] Dobrez DG, Mathes A, Amdahl M, Marx SE, *et al.* Paricalcitol-treated patients experience improved hospitalization outcomes compared with calcitriol-treated patients in real-world clinical settings. *Nephrol Dial Transplant* 2004; 19: 1174-1181.

[55] Marco MP, Craver L, Betriu A, Fibla J, *et al.* Influence of vitamin D receptor gene polymorphisms on mortality risk in hemodialysis patients. *Am J Kidney Dis* 2001; 38: 965-974.

[56] Kalantar-Zadeh K, Kuwae N, Regidor DL, Kovesdy CP, *et al.* Survival predictability of time-varying indicators of bone disease in maintenance hemodialysis patients. *Kidney Int* 2006; 70: 771-780.

[57] Wolf M, Shah A, Gutierrez O, Ankers E, *et al.* Vitamin D levels and early mortality among incident hemodialysis patients. *Kidney Int* 2007; 72: 1004-1013.

[58] Teng M, Wolf M, Ofsthun MN, Lazarus JM, *et al.* Activated injectable vitamin D and hemodialysis survival: a historical cohort study. *J Am Soc Nephrol* 2005; 16: 1115-1125.

[59] Naves-Diaz M, Alvarez-Hernandez D, Passlick-Deetjen J, Guinsburg A, *et al.* Oral active vitamin D is associated with improved survival in hemodialysis patients. *Kidney Int* 2008; 74: 1070-1078.

[60] Shoji T, Shinohara K, Kimoto E, Emoto M, *et al.* Lower risk for cardiovascular mortality in oral 1alpha-hydroxy vitamin D3 users in a haemodialysis population. *Nephrol Dial Transplant* 2004; 19: 179-184.

[61] Kovesdy CP, Ahmadzadeh S, Anderson JE, Kalantar-Zadeh K. Association of activated vitamin D treatment and mortality in chronic kidney disease. *Arch Intern Med* 2008; 168: 397-403.

[62] Shoben AB, Rudser KD, de Boer IH, Young B, *et al.* Association of oral calcitriol with improved survival in nondialyzed CKD. *J Am Soc Nephrol* 2008; 19: 1613-1619.

[63] Melamed ML, Michos ED, Post W, Astor B. 25-hydroxyvitamin D levels and the risk of mortality in the general population. *Arch Intern Med* 2008; 168: 1629-1637.

[64] Tentori F. Focus on vitamin D therapy in chronic kidney disease. *J Nephrol* 2007; 20: 511-514.

[65] Holick MF. Vitamin D: A millenium perspective. *J Cell Biochem* 2003; 88: 296-307.

[66] Nagpal S, Na S, Rathnachalam R. Noncalcemic actions of vitamin D receptor ligands. *Endocr Rev* 2005; 26: 662-687.
[67] Eleftheriadis T, Antoniadi G, Liakopoulos V, Kartsios C, *et al.* Disturbances of acquired immunity in hemodialysis patients. *Semin Dial* 2007; 20: 440-451.
[68] Patsalas S, Eleftheriadis T, Spaia S, Theodoroglou H, *et al.* Thirty-month follow-up of coronary artery calcification in hemodialysis patients: different roles for inflammation and abnormal calcium-phosphorous metabolism? *Ren Fail* 2007; 29: 623-629.
[69] Zimmermann J, Herrlinger S, Pruy A, Metzger T, *et al.* Inflammation enhances cardiovascular risk and mortality in hemodialysis patients. *Kidney Int* 1999; 55: 648-658.
[70] Stenvinkel P, Heimburger O, Lindholm B, Kaysen GA, *et al.* Are there two types of malnutrition in chronic renal failure? Evidence for relationships between malnutrition, inflammation and atherosclerosis (MIA syndrome). *Nephrol Dial Transplant* 2000; 15: 953-960.
[71] Eleftheriadis T, Kartsios C, Yiannaki E, Kazila P, *et al.* Chronic inflammation and T cell zeta-chain downregulation in hemodialysis patients. *Am J Nephrol* 2008; 28: 152-157.
[72] Eleftheriadis T, Kartsios C, Yiannaki E, Kazila P, *et al.* Chronic inflammation and CD16+ natural killer cell zeta-chain downregulation in hemodialysis patients. *Blood Purif* 2008; 26: 317-321.
[73] Sarnak MJ, Jaber BL. Mortality caused by sepsis in patients with end-stage renal disease compared with the general population. *Kidney Int* 2000; 58: 1758-1764.
[74] van Dijk PC, Jager KJ, de Charro F, Collart F, *et al.* Renal replacement therapy in Europe: the results of a collaborative effort by the ERA-EDTA registry and six national or regional registries. *Nephrol Dial Transplant* 2001; 16: 1120-1129.
[75] Steketee RW, Ziarnik ME, Davis JP. Seroresponse to hepatitis B vaccine in patients and staff of renal dialysis centers, Wisconsin. *Am J Epidemiol* 1988; 127: 772-782.
[76] Kohler H, Arnold W, Renschin G, Dormeyer HH, *et al.* Active hepatitis B vaccination of dialysis patients and medical staff. *Kidney Int* 1984; 25: 124-128.
[77] Stevens CE, Alter HJ, Taylor PE, Zang EA, *et al.* Hepatitis B vaccine in patients receiving hemodialysis. Immunogenicity and efficacy. *N Engl J Med* 1984; 311: 496-501.

[78] Eleftheriadis T, Kartsios C, Liakopoulos V, Antoniadi G, *et al.* Does hepcidin affect erythropoiesis in hemodialysis patients? *Acta Haematol* 2006; 116: 238-244.

[79] Eleftheriadis T, Liakopoulos V, Antoniadi G, Kartsios C, *et al.* The role of hepcidin in iron homeostasis and anemia in hemodialysis patients. *Semin Dial* 2009; 22: 70-77.

[80] Ravani P, Malberti F, Tripepi G, Pecchini P, *et al.* Vitamin D levels and patient outcome in chronic kidney disease. *Kidney Int* 2009; 75: 88-95.

[81] Agarwal R, Acharya M, Tian J, Hippensteel RL, *et al.* Antiproteinuric effect of oral paricalcitol in chronic kidney disease. *Kidney Int* 2005; 68: 2823-2828.

[82] Provvedini DM, Tsoukas CD, Deftos LJ, Manolagas SC. 1,25-dihydroxyvitamin D3 receptors in human leukocytes. *Science* 1983; 221: 1181-1183.

[83] Rigby WF, Stacy T, Fanger MW. Inhibition of T lymphocyte mitogenesis by 1,25-dihydroxyvitamin D3 (calcitriol). *J Clin Invest* 1984; 74: 1451-1455.

[84] Rigby WF, Denome S, Fanger MW. Regulation of lymphokine production and human T lymphocyte activation by 1,25-dihydroxyvitamin D3. Specific inhibition at the level of messenger RNA. *J Clin Invest* 1987; 79: 1659-1664.

[85] Mahon BD, Wittke A, Weaver V, Cantorna MT. The targets of vitamin D depend on the differentiation and activation status of CD4 positive T cells. *J Cell Biochem* 2003; 89: 922-932.

[86] Adams JS, Sharma OP, Gacad MA, Singer FR. Metabolism of 25-hydroxyvitamin D3 by cultured pulmonary alveolar macrophages in sarcoidosis. *J Clin Invest* 1983; 72: 1856-1860.

[87] Monkawa T, Yoshida T, Hayashi M, Saruta T. Identification of 25-hydroxyvitamin D3 1alpha-hydroxylase gene expression in macrophages. *Kidney Int* 2000; 58: 559-568.

[88] Fritsche J, Mondal K, Ehrnsperger A, Andreesen R, *et al.* Regulation of 25-hydroxyvitamin D3-1 alpha-hydroxylase and production of 1 alpha,25-dihydroxyvitamin D3 by human dendritic cells. *Blood* 2003; 102: 3314-3316.

[89] Liu PT, Stenger S, Li H, Wenzel L, *et al.* Toll-like receptor triggering of a vitamin D-mediated human antimicrobial response. *Science* 2006; 311: 1770-1773.

[90] Overbergh L, Decallonne B, Valckx D, Verstuyf A, *et al.* Identification and immune regulation of 25-hydroxyvitamin D-1-alpha-

hydroxylase in murine macrophages. *Clin Exp Immunol* 2000; 120: 139-146.

[91] Hewison M, Freeman L, Hughes SV, Evans KN, *et al.* Differential regulation of vitamin D receptor and its ligand in human monocyte-derived dendritic cells. *J Immunol* 2003; 170: 5382-5390.

[92] Cantorna MT, Munsick C, Bemiss C, Mahon BD. 1,25-Dihydroxycholecalciferol prevents and ameliorates symptoms of experimental murine inflammatory bowel disease. *J Nutr* 2000; 130: 2648-2652.

[93] Froicu M, Weaver V, Wynn TA, McDowell MA, *et al.* A crucial role for the vitamin D receptor in experimental inflammatory bowel diseases. *Mol Endocrinol* 2003; 17: 2386-2392.

[94] Lemire JM, Archer DC. 1,25-dihydroxyvitamin D3 prevents the in vivo induction of murine experimental autoimmune encephalomyelitis. *J Clin Invest* 1991; 87: 1103-1107.

[95] Abe J, Nakamura K, Takita Y, Nakano T, *et al.* Prevention of immunological disorders in MRL/l mice by a new synthetic analogue of vitamin D3: 22-oxa-1 alpha,25-dihydroxyvitamin D3. *J Nutr Sci Vitaminol (Tokyo)* 1990; 36: 21-31.

[96] Lemire JM, Ince A, Takashima M. 1,25-Dihydroxyvitamin D3 attenuates the expression of experimental murine lupus of MRL/l mice. *Autoimmunity* 1992; 12: 143-148.

[97] Mathieu C, Waer M, Laureys J, Rutgeerts O, *et al.* Prevention of autoimmune diabetes in NOD mice by 1,25 dihydroxyvitamin D3. *Diabetologia* 1994; 37: 552-558.

[98] Gregori S, Giarratana N, Smiroldo S, Uskokovic M, *et al.* A 1alpha,25-dihydroxyvitamin D(3) analog enhances regulatory T-cells and arrests autoimmune diabetes in NOD mice. *Diabetes* 2002; 51: 1367-1374.

[99] Larsson P, Mattsson L, Klareskog L, Johnsson C. A vitamin D analogue (MC 1288) has immunomodulatory properties and suppresses collagen-induced arthritis (CIA) without causing hypercalcaemia. *Clin Exp Immunol* 1998; 114: 277-283.

[100] Branisteanu DD, Leenaerts P, van Damme B, Bouillon R. Partial prevention of active Heymann nephritis by 1 alpha, 25 dihydroxyvitamin D3. *Clin Exp Immunol* 1993; 94: 412-417.

[101] Redaelli CA, Wagner M, Gunter-Duwe D, Tian YH, *et al.* 1alpha,25-dihydroxyvitamin D3 shows strong and additive immunomodulatory effects with cyclosporine A in rat renal allotransplants. *Kidney Int* 2002; 61: 288-296.

[102] Redaelli CA, Wagner M, Tien YH, Mazzucchelli L, *et al.* 1 alpha,25-Dihydroxycholecalciferol reduces rejection and improves survival in rat liver allografts. *Hepatology* 2001; 34: 926-934.
[103] Gregori S, Casorati M, Amuchastegui S, Smiroldo S, *et al.* Regulatory T cells induced by 1 alpha,25-dihydroxyvitamin D3 and mycophenolate mofetil treatment mediate transplantation tolerance. *J Immunol* 2001; 167: 1945-1953.
[104] Hullett DA, Cantorna MT, Redaelli C, Humpal-Winter J, *et al.* Prolongation of allograft survival by 1,25-dihydroxyvitamin D3. *Transplantation* 1998; 66: 824-828.
[105] Raisanen-Sokolowski AK, Pakkala IS, Samila SP, Binderup L, *et al.* A vitamin D analog, MC1288, inhibits adventitial inflammation and suppresses intimal lesions in rat aortic allografts. *Transplantation* 1997; 63: 936-941.
[106] van Etten E, Branisteanu DD, Verstuyf A, Waer M, *et al.* Analogs of 1,25-dihydroxyvitamin D3 as dose-reducing agents for classical immunosuppressants. *Transplantation* 2000; 69: 1932-1942.
[107] Mathieu C, Waer M, Laureys J, Rutgeerts O, *et al.* Activated form of vitamin D [1,25(OH)2D3] and its analogs are dose-reducing agents for cyclosporine in vitro and in vivo. *Transplant Proc* 1994; 26: 3048-3049.
[108] Mathieu C, Laureys J, Waer M, Bouillon R. Prevention of autoimmune destruction of transplanted islets in spontaneously diabetic NOD mice by KH1060, a 20-epi analog of vitamin D: synergy with cyclosporine. *Transplant Proc* 1994; 26: 3128-3129.
[109] Mathieu C, Bouillon R, Rutgeerts O, Vandeputte M, *et al.* Potential role of 1,25(OH)2 vitamin D3 as a dose-reducing agent for cyclosporine and FK 506. *Transplant Proc* 1994; 26: 3130.
[110] Cantorna MT, Hullett DA, Redaelli C, Brandt CR, *et al.* 1,25-Dihydroxyvitamin D3 prolongs graft survival without compromising host resistance to infection or bone mineral density. *Transplantation* 1998; 66: 828-831.
[111] Ustianowski A, Shaffer R, Collin S, Wilkinson RJ, *et al.* Prevalence and associations of vitamin D deficiency in foreign-born persons with tuberculosis in London. *J Infect* 2005; 50: 432-437.
[112] Liu PT, Krutzik SR, Modlin RL. Therapeutic implications of the TLR and VDR partnership. *Trends Mol Med* 2007; 13: 117-124.
[113] Gombart AF, Borregaard N, Koeffler HP. Human cathelicidin antimicrobial peptide (CAMP) gene is a direct target of the vitamin D

receptor and is strongly up-regulated in myeloid cells by 1,25-dihydroxyvitamin D3. *FASEB J* 2005; 19: 1067-1077.

[114] Jahnsen J, Falch JA, Mowinckel P, Aadland E. Vitamin D status, parathyroid hormone and bone mineral density in patients with inflammatory bowel disease. *Scand J Gastroenterol* 2002; 37: 192-199.

[115] Lamb EJ, Wong T, Smith DJ, Simpson DE, *et al.* Metabolic bone disease is present at diagnosis in patients with inflammatory bowel disease. *Aliment Pharmacol Ther* 2002; 16: 1895-1902.

[116] Nieves J, Cosman F, Herbert J, Shen V, *et al.* High prevalence of vitamin D deficiency and reduced bone mass in multiple sclerosis. *Neurology* 1994; 44: 1687-1692.

[117] Munger KL, Zhang SM, O'Reilly E, Hernan MA, *et al.* Vitamin D intake and incidence of multiple sclerosis. *Neurology* 2004; 62: 60-65.

[118] Munger KL, Levin LI, Hollis BW, Howard NS, *et al.* Serum 25-hydroxyvitamin D levels and risk of multiple sclerosis. *JAMA* 2006; 296: 2832-2838.

[119] Kamen DL, Cooper GS, Bouali H, Shaftman SR, *et al.* Vitamin D deficiency in systemic lupus erythematosus. *Autoimmun Rev* 2006; 5: 114-117.

[120] Vitamin D supplement in early childhood and risk for Type I (insulin-dependent) diabetes mellitus. The EURODIAB Substudy 2 Study Group. *Diabetologia* 1999; 42: 51-54.

[121] Hypponen E, Laara E, Reunanen A, Jarvelin MR, *et al.* Intake of vitamin D and risk of type 1 diabetes: a birth-cohort study. *Lancet* 2001; 358: 1500-1503.

[122] Andjelkovic Z, Vojinovic J, Pejnovic N, Popovic M, *et al.* Disease modifying and immunomodulatory effects of high dose 1 alpha (OH) D3 in rheumatoid arthritis patients. *Clin Exp Rheumatol* 1999; 17: 453-456.

[123] P, del Campo MT, Garces MV, Gonzalez-Casaus ML, *et al.* Low vitamin D levels in outpatient postmenopausal women from a rheumatology clinic in Madrid, Spain: their relationship with bone mineral density. *Osteoporos Int* 2000; 11: 739-744.

[124] Merlino LA, Curtis J, Mikuls TR, Cerhan JR, *et al.* Vitamin D intake is inversely associated with rheumatoid arthritis: results from the Iowa Women's Health Study. *Arthritis Rheum* 2004; 50: 72-77.

[125] Chan TY. Vitamin D deficiency and susceptibility to tuberculosis. *Calcif Tissue Int* 2000; 66: 476-478.

[126] Timms PM, Mannan N, Hitman GA, Noonan K, *et al.* Circulating MMP9, vitamin D and variation in the TIMP-1 response with VDR

genotype: mechanisms for inflammatory damage in chronic disorders? *QJM* 2002; 95: 787-796.

[127] Gannage-Yared MH, Azoury M, Mansour I, Baddoura R, *et al.* Effects of a short-term calcium and vitamin D treatment on serum cytokines, bone markers, insulin and lipid concentrations in healthy post-menopausal women. *J Endocrinol Invest* 2003; 26: 748-753.

[128] Griffin MD, Lutz W, Phan VA, Bachman LA, *et al.* Dendritic cell modulation by 1alpha,25 dihydroxyvitamin D3 and its analogs: a vitamin D receptor-dependent pathway that promotes a persistent state of immaturity in vitro and in vivo. *Proc Natl Acad Sci U S A* 2001; 98: 6800-6805.

[129] Penna G, Adorini L. 1 Alpha,25-dihydroxyvitamin D3 inhibits differentiation, maturation, activation, and survival of dendritic cells leading to impaired alloreactive T cell activation. *J Immunol* 2000; 164: 2405-2411.

[130] D'Ambrosio D, Cippitelli M, Cocciolo MG, Mazzeo D, *et al.* Inhibition of IL-12 production by 1,25-dihydroxyvitamin D3. Involvement of NF-kappaB downregulation in transcriptional repression of the p40 gene. *J Clin Invest* 1998; 101: 252-262.

[131] Lemire JM, Archer DC, Beck L, Spiegelberg HL. Immunosuppressive actions of 1,25-dihydroxyvitamin D3: preferential inhibition of Th1 functions. *J Nutr* 1995; 125: 1704S-1708S.

[132] Boonstra A, Barrat FJ, Crain C, Heath VL, *et al.* 1alpha,25-Dihydroxyvitamin d3 has a direct effect on naive CD4(+) T cells to enhance the development of Th2 cells. *J Immunol* 2001; 167: 4974-4980.

[133] Daniel C, Sartory NA, Zahn N, Radeke HH, *et al.* Immune modulatory treatment of trinitrobenzene sulfonic acid colitis with calcitriol is associated with a change of a T helper (Th) 1/Th17 to a Th2 and regulatory T cell profile. *J Pharmacol Exp Ther* 2008; 324: 23-33.

[134] Chen S, Sims GP, Chen XX, Gu YY, *et al.* Modulatory effects of 1,25-dihydroxyvitamin D3 on human B cell differentiation. *J Immunol* 2007; 179: 1634-1647.

[135] Linker-Israeli M, Elstner E, Klinenberg JR, Wallace DJ, *et al.* Vitamin D(3) and its synthetic analogs inhibit the spontaneous in vitro immunoglobulin production by SLE-derived PBMC. *Clin Immunol* 2001; 99: 82-93.

[136] Helming L, Bose J, Ehrchen J, Schiebe S, *et al.* 1alpha,25-Dihydroxyvitamin D3 is a potent suppressor of interferon gamma-mediated macrophage activation. *Blood* 2005; 106: 4351-4358.
[137] Abu-Amer Y, Bar-Shavit Z. Regulation of TNF-alpha release from bone marrow-derived macrophages by vitamin D. *J Cell Biochem* 1994; 55: 435-444.
[138] Tabata T, Shoji T, Kikunami K, Matsushita Y, *et al.* In vivo effect of 1 alpha-hydroxyvitamin D3 on interleukin-2 production in hemodialysis patients. *Nephron* 1988; 50: 295-298.
[139] Riancho JA, Zarrabeitia MT, de Francisco AL, Amado JA, *et al.* Vitamin D therapy modulates cytokine secretion in patients with renal failure. *Nephron* 1993; 65: 364-368.
[140] Antonen J, Saha H, Lagerstedt A, Krohn K, *et al.* Intravenous calcitriol therapy restores reduced antigen-induced T-lymphocyte response in 1,25-(OH)2D3-deficient hemodialysis patients. *Nephron* 1996; 74: 680-686.
[141] Turk S, Akbulut M, Yildiz A, Gurbilek M, *et al.* Comparative effect of oral pulse and intravenous calcitriol treatment in hemodialysis patients: the effect on serum IL-1 and IL-6 levels and bone mineral density. *Nephron* 2002; 90: 188-194.
[142] Eleftheriadis T, Antoniadi G, Liakopoulos V, Kartsios C, *et al.* Paricalcitol reduces basal and lipopolysaccharide-induced (LPS) TNF-alpha and IL-8 production by human peripheral blood mononuclear cells. *Int Urol Nephrol* 2009. (DOI: 10.1007/s11255-009-9541-1)
[143] Eleftheriadis T, Antoniadi G, Liakopoulos V, Galaktidou G. The effect of paricalcitol on osteoprotegerin production by human peripheral blood mononuclear cells. *J Rheumatol* 2009; 36: 856-857.
[144] Li Y, Toraldo G, Li A, Yang X, *et al.* B cells and T cells are critical for the preservation of bone homeostasis and attainment of peak bone mass in vivo. *Blood* 2007; 109: 3839-3848.
[145] Alborzi P, Patel NA, Peterson C, Bills JE, *et al.* Paricalcitol reduces albuminuria and inflammation in chronic kidney disease: a randomized double-blind pilot trial. *Hypertension* 2008; 52: 249-255.
[146] Tan X, Wen X, Liu Y. Paricalcitol inhibits renal inflammation by promoting vitamin D receptor-mediated sequestration of NF-kappaB signaling. *J Am Soc Nephrol* 2008; 19: 1741-1752.
[147] Del Valle E, Negri AL, Aguirre C, Fradinger E, *et al.* Prevalence of 25(OH) vitamin D insufficiency and deficiency in chronic kidney

disease stage 5 patients on hemodialysis. *Hemodial Int* 2007; 11: 315-321.

[148] Gomez-Alonso C, Naves-Diaz ML, Fernandez-Martin JL, Diaz-Lopez JB, *et al.* Vitamin D status and secondary hyperparathyroidism: the importance of 25-hydroxyvitamin D cut-off levels. *Kidney Int Suppl* 2003: S44-48.

[149] Holick MF. Vitamin D deficiency. *N Engl J Med* 2007; 357: 266-281.

[150] Holick MF. Resurrection of vitamin D deficiency and rickets. *J Clin Invest* 2006; 116: 2062-2072.

[151] Kisseleva T, Brenner DA. Mechanisms of fibrogenesis. *Exp Biol Med (Maywood)* 2008; 233: 109-122.

[152] Sivakumar P, Das AM. Fibrosis, chronic inflammation and new pathways for drug discovery. *Inflamm Res* 2008; 57: 410-418.

[153] Broughton G, 2nd, Janis JE, Attinger CE. The basic science of wound healing. *Plast Reconstr Surg* 2006; 117: 12S-34S.

[154] Darby IA, Hewitson TD. Fibroblast differentiation in wound healing and fibrosis. *Int Rev Cytol* 2007; 257: 143-179.

[155] Hinz B, Phan SH, Thannickal VJ, Galli A, *et al.* The myofibroblast: one function, multiple origins. *Am J Pathol* 2007; 170: 1807-1816.

[156] Prud'homme GJ. Pathobiology of transforming growth factor beta in cancer, fibrosis and immunologic disease, and therapeutic considerations. *Lab Invest* 2007; 87: 1077-1091.

[157] Sheppard D. Integrin-mediated activation of latent transforming growth factor beta. *Cancer Metastasis Rev* 2005; 24: 395-402.

[158] Massague J. How cells read TGF-beta signals. *Nat Rev Mol Cell Biol* 2000; 1: 169-178.

[159] Schmierer B, Hill CS. TGFbeta-SMAD signal transduction: molecular specificity and functional flexibility. *Nat Rev Mol Cell Biol* 2007; 8: 970-982.

[160] Gressner OA, Gressner AM. Connective tissue growth factor: a fibrogenic master switch in fibrotic liver diseases. *Liver Int* 2008; 28: 1065-1079.

[161] Park SH. Fine tuning and cross-talking of TGF-beta signal by inhibitory Smads. *J Biochem Mol Biol* 2005; 38: 9-16.

[162] Zhang YE. Non-Smad pathways in TGF-beta signaling. *Cell Res* 2009; 19: 128-139.

[163] Wang W, Koka V, Lan HY. Transforming growth factor-beta and Smad signalling in kidney diseases. *Nephrology (Carlton)* 2005; 10: 48-56.

[164] Kagami S, Border WA, Miller DE, Noble NA. Angiotensin II stimulates extracellular matrix protein synthesis through induction of transforming growth factor-beta expression in rat glomerular mesangial cells. *J Clin Invest* 1994; 93: 2431-2437.
[165] Huang Y, Wongamorntham S, Kasting J, McQuillan D, *et al.* Renin increases mesangial cell transforming growth factor-beta1 and matrix proteins through receptor-mediated, angiotensin II-independent mechanisms. *Kidney Int* 2006; 69: 105-113.
[166] Hirata M, Makibayashi K, Katsumata K, Kusano K, *et al.* 22-Oxacalcitriol prevents progressive glomerulosclerosis without adversely affecting calcium and phosphorus metabolism in subtotally nephrectomized rats. *Nephrol Dial Transplant* 2002; 17: 2132-2137.
[167] Schwarz U, Amann K, Orth SR, Simonaviciene A, *et al.* Effect of 1,25 (OH)2 vitamin D3 on glomerulosclerosis in subtotally nephrectomized rats. *Kidney Int* 1998; 53: 1696-1705.
[168] Sanai T, Tokumoto M, Hirano T, Okuda S. Different effects of 22-oxacalcitriol and calcitriol on the course of experimental chronic renal failure. *J Lab Clin Med* 2002; 140: 242-249.
[169] Kuhlmann A, Haas CS, Gross ML, Reulbach U, *et al.* 1,25-Dihydroxyvitamin D3 decreases podocyte loss and podocyte hypertrophy in the subtotally nephrectomized rat. *Am J Physiol Renal Physiol* 2004; 286: F526-533.
[170] Eddy AA. Molecular basis of renal fibrosis. *Pediatr Nephrol* 2000; 15: 290-301.
[171] Liu Y. Renal fibrosis: new insights into the pathogenesis and therapeutics. *Kidney Int* 2006; 69: 213-217.
[172] Rastaldi MP, Ferrario F, Giardino L, Dell'Antonio G, *et al.* Epithelial-mesenchymal transition of tubular epithelial cells in human renal biopsies. *Kidney Int* 2002; 62: 137-146.
[173] Poulsom R, Forbes SJ, Hodivala-Dilke K, Ryan E, *et al.* Bone marrow contributes to renal parenchymal turnover and regeneration. *J Pathol* 2001; 195: 229-235.
[174] Iwano M, Plieth D, Danoff TM, Xue C, *et al.* Evidence that fibroblasts derive from epithelium during tissue fibrosis. *J Clin Invest* 2002; 110: 341-350.
[175] Hay ED, Zuk A. Transformations between epithelium and mesenchyme: normal, pathological, and experimentally induced. *Am J Kidney Dis* 1995; 26: 678-690.

[176] Sato M, Muragaki Y, Saika S, Roberts AB, *et al.* Targeted disruption of TGF-beta1/Smad3 signaling protects against renal tubulointerstitial fibrosis induced by unilateral ureteral obstruction. *J Clin Invest* 2003; 112: 1486-1494.

[177] Tan X, Li Y, Liu Y. Paricalcitol attenuates renal interstitial fibrosis in obstructive nephropathy. *J Am Soc Nephrol* 2006; 17: 3382-3393.

[178] Aschenbrenner JK, Sollinger HW, Becker BN, Hullett DA. 1,25-(OH(2))D(3) alters the transforming growth factor beta signaling pathway in renal tissue. *J Surg Res* 2001; 100: 171-175.

[179] Yanagisawa J, Yanagi Y, Masuhiro Y, Suzawa M, *et al.* Convergence of transforming growth factor-beta and vitamin D signaling pathways on SMAD transcriptional coactivators. *Science* 1999; 283: 1317-1321.

[180] Gupta S, Clarkson MR, Duggan J, Brady HR. Connective tissue growth factor: potential role in glomerulosclerosis and tubulointerstitial fibrosis. *Kidney Int* 2000; 58: 1389-1399.

[181] Mizobuchi M, Morrissey J, Finch JL, Martin DR, *et al.* Combination therapy with an angiotensin-converting enzyme inhibitor and a vitamin D analog suppresses the progression of renal insufficiency in uremic rats. *J Am Soc Nephrol* 2007; 18: 1796-1806.

[182] Li YC, Kong J, Wei M, Chen ZF, *et al.* 1,25-Dihydroxyvitamin D(3) is a negative endocrine regulator of the renin-angiotensin system. *J Clin Invest* 2002; 110: 229-238.

[183] Freundlich M, Quiroz Y, Zhang Z, Zhang Y, *et al.* Suppression of renin-angiotensin gene expression in the kidney by paricalcitol. *Kidney Int* 2008; 74: 1394-1402.

[184] W, Kong J, Chen S, Cao LP, *et al.* Cardiac hypertrophy in vitamin D receptor knockout mice: role of the systemic and cardiac renin-angiotensin systems. *Am J Physiol Endocrinol Metab* 2005; 288: E125-132.

[185] Pan L, Black TA, Shi Q, Jones CA, *et al.* Critical roles of a cyclic AMP responsive element and an E-box in regulation of mouse renin gene expression. *J Biol Chem* 2001; 276: 45530-45538.

[186] Zhang Z, Sun L, Wang Y, Ning G, *et al.* Renoprotective role of the vitamin D receptor in diabetic nephropathy. *Kidney Int* 2008; 73: 163-171.

[187] Zhang Z, Zhang Y, Ning G, Deb DK, *et al.* Combination therapy with AT1 blocker and vitamin D analog markedly ameliorates diabetic nephropathy: blockade of compensatory renin increase. *Proc Natl Acad Sci U S A* 2008; 105: 15896-15901.

In: Vitamin D: Biochemistry, Nutrition ... ISBN: 978-1-61668-273-6
Editor: W. J. Stackhouse, pp. 67-103

Chapter 3

VITAMIN D DEFICIENCY AND ITS HEALTH CONSEQUENCES

***Diana Badiu**[*1] **and Rafael Luque**[‡2]*
[1]Ovidius University of Constanta, Constanta, Romania
[2]Universidad de Cordoba, Campus de Rabanales
Edificio Marie Curie, Cordoba, Spain

ABSTRACT

Vitamin D is a group of liposoluble components that organisms can obtain either via endogenous production from sun exposure or directly taken from foods and dietary supplements. In addition to its involvement in calcium metabolism, its presence plays other important functions in human health (e.g. reduction of inflammation and effects on cell proliferation and differentiation).

The discovery that most tissues and cells in the body have a vitamin D receptor and that several possess the enzymatic machinery to convert the primary circulating form of vitamin D (25-hydroxycholecalciferol, hydroxylated vitamin D3) to the active form (1,25-dihydroxycholecalciferol, calcitriol) has provided new insights into the

* Department of Biochemistry, Faculty of Natural and Agricultural Sciences, Ovidius University of Constanta, 124, Mamaia Blvd., 900527 Constanta, Romania, E-mail: dianabadiu@yahoo.com

‡ Departamento de Quimica Organica, Universidad de CordobaCampus de Rabanales, Edificio Marie Curie (C-3) Ctra Nnal IV, Km 396, Cordoba (Spain), E-14014, E-mail: q62alsor@uco.es

function of this vitamin. Of great interest is the role it can play in decreasing the risk of many chronic illnesses, including common autoimmune diseases, cardiovascular disease, and cancers among others.

This chapter reviews the nature of vitamin D deficiency, its causes and effects on the human organism, and suggest strategies for its prevention and treatment by both natural sources and/or vitamin D supplements.

Key words: 1,25-hydroxyvitamin D_3, vitamin D receptor, metabolism, deficiency, treatment.

1. Sources, Types and Metabolism of Vitamin D

Vitamin D, known as the "sunshine vitamin", has been taken for granted and, until recently, little attention has been focused on its important role for adult bone health and for prevention of many chronic diseases. It has been assumed that vitamin D deficiency is no longer a health issue in the United States and Europe. However, it is now recognized that everyone is at risk for vitamin D deficiency (Holick, 1989).

Although it is not known when vitamin D was first made on Earth, it has been demonstrated that a phytoplankton species *Emiliani huxleii*, which has existed unchanged in the Atlantic Ocean for more than 750 million years, has the ability, when exposed to sunlight, to make vitamin D (Holick, 1989). As life forms evolved in the oceans, they took advantage of its high calcium content and used it as a mediator for a variety of metabolic functions, as well as for controlling neuromuscular activity. As vertebrate evolved, they found the ocean environment to be plentiful in calcium and therefore could take out of their environment the calcium required for a healthy mineralized skeleton. However, when vertebrates ventured onto the land masses, they needed to make vitamin D to enhance the efficiency of calcium absorption (Holick, 2003).

During exposure to sunlight, ultraviolet B (UVB) photons (290-315 nm) penetrate into the viable epidermis and dermis where they are absorbed by 7-dehydrocholesterol that is present in the plasma membrane of these cells. Figure 1 present synthesis and metabolism of vitamin D in the regulation of calcium, phosphorus, and bone metabolism. The absorption of UVB radiation causes 7-dehydrocholesterol to open its B ring, forming precholecalciferol. Precholecalciferol is inherently unstable and rapidly undergoes rearrangement of its double bonds to form cholecalciferol (vitamin D_3). As cholecalciferol is being formed, it is ejected out of the plasma membrane into the extracellular space, where it enters into the dermal capillary bed, drawn in by the vitamin D binding protein (DBP) (Holick, 2003).

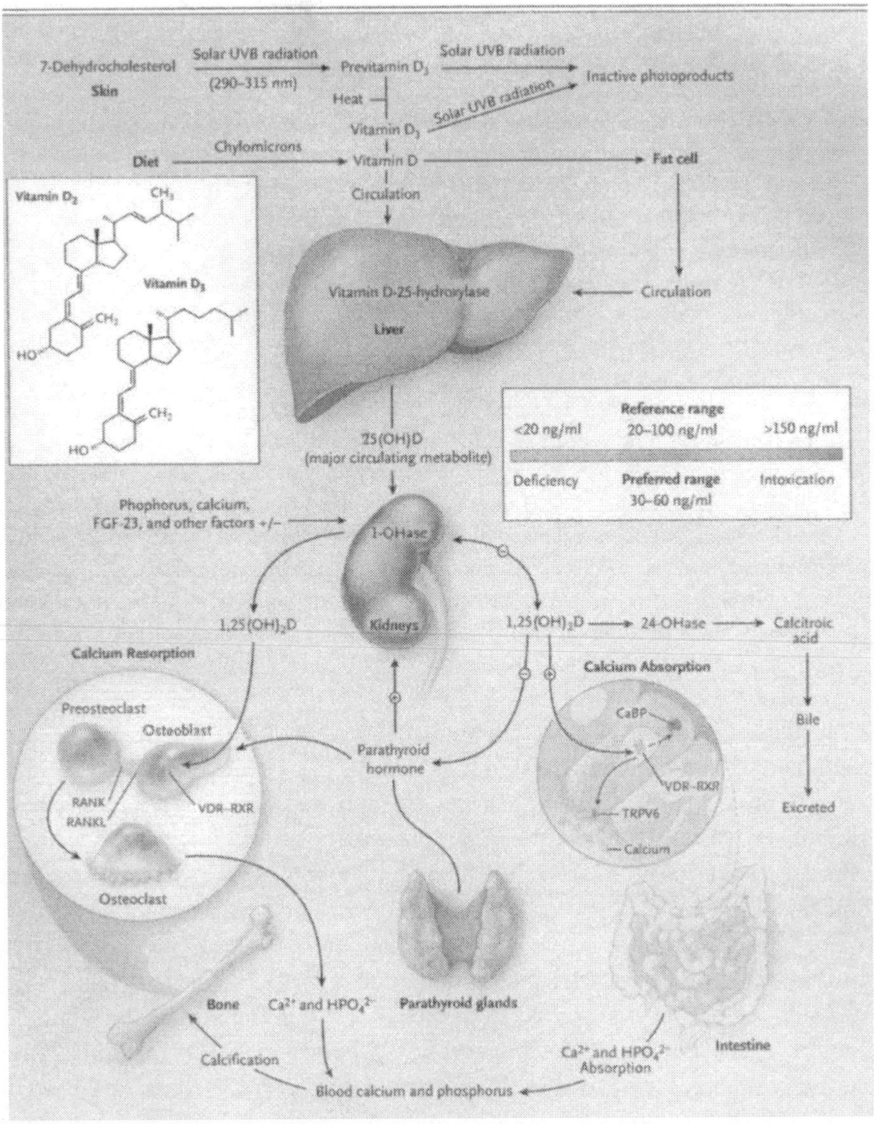

Figure 1. Synthesis and metabolism of vitamin D in the regulation of calcium, phosphorus, and bone metabolism.

Legend. During exposure to solar UVB radiation, 7-dehydrocholesterol in the skin is converted to previtamin D_3, which is immediately converted to vitamin D_3 in a heat-dependent process. Excessive exposure to sunlight degrades previtamin D_3 and vitamin D_3 into inactive photoproducts. Vitamin D_2 and vitamin D_3 from dietary sources are incorporated into chylomicrons and transported by the limphatic system into the venous circulation. Vitamin D (hereafter „D" represents D_2 or D_3) made in the skin or ingested in the diet can be stored in and then released from fat cells. Vitamin D in the circulation is bound to the DBP, which transports it to the liver, where vitamin D-25-hydroxylase to $25(OH)D_3$. This is the major circulating form of vitamin D that is used by clinicians to determine vitamin D status (although most laboratories report the normal range to be 20 to 100 ng per milliliter, the prefered ranged is 30 to 60 ng per milliliter). This form of vitamin D is biologically inactive and must be converted in the kidneys by $25(OH)D_3$-1α-hydroxylase to the biologically active form, $1,25(OH)_2D_3$. Serum phosphorus, calcium, fibroblast growth factor 23, and other factors can either increase or decrease the renal production of $1,25(OH)_2D_3$. $1,25(OH)_2D_3$ enhances intestinal calcium absorption in the small intestine by interacting with the VDR-retinoic acid x-receptor complex to enhance the expression of the epithelial channel and calbindin 9K, a calcium-BP. $1,25(OH)_2D_3$ is recognized by its receptor in osteoblasts, causing an increase in the expression of the receptor activator of nuclear factor-k B ligand. The receptor from preosteoclasts binds this factor which induces preosteoclasts to become mature osteoclasts. Mature osteoclasts remove calcium and phosphorus from the bone, maintaining calcium and phosphorus levels in the blood. Adequate calcium (Ca^{2+}) and phosphorus (HPO_4^{2-}) levels promote the mineralization of the skeleton (adapted from Folick, 2007).

It was suggested that skin pigmentation evolved to prevent excess production of vitamin D in the skin (Loomis, 1970). However, there was never been a reported case of vitamin D intoxication due to excessive exposure to sunlight for white lifeguards and sun worshippers or for tanners who frequent a tanning salon. The reason for this is that when precholecalciferol and cholecalciferol are exposed to sunlight, they undergo transformation of their double bonds to form a wide variety of photoisomers that have little biologic actitivity on calcium metabolism (Holick *et al.*, 1981).

Once vitamin D is absorbed from diet or made in the skin by the action of sunlight, it is metabolized in the liver to 25-hydroxyvitamin D_3 [$25(OH)D_3$] and then in the kidney to 1,25-dihydroxyvitamin D_3 [$1,25(OH)_2D_3$], the active form. $1,25(OH)_2D_3$ interacts with its nuclear receptor (VDR) in the intestine and bone in order to maintain calcium homeostasis. The VDR is also present in a wide variety of other tissues. $1,25(OH)_2D_3$ interacts with these receptors to have a multitude of important physiological effects. In addition, it is now recognized that many tissues, including colon, breast and prostate, have the enzymatic machinery to produce $1,25(OH)_2D_3$. The insights into the new biological functions of $1,25(OH)_2D_3$ in regulating cell growth, modulating the immune system and the rennin-angiotensin system provides an explanation for why diminished sun exposure at higher latitudes is associated with increased risk of dying of many common cancers, developing type 1 diabetes and multiple sclerosis (MS), and having a higher incidence of hypertension (Holick, 2003).

Few foods naturally contain or are fortified with vitamin D. The "D" represents D_2 or D_3. Vitamin D_2 (ergocalciferol) is manufactured through the UV irradiation of ergosterol from yeast, and vitamin D_3 through the ultraviolet irradiation of 7-dehydrocholesterol from lanolin. Both are used in over-the-counter vitamin D supplements, but the form available by prescription in the United States is vitamin D_2 (Krause *et al.*, 1998).

Vitamin D (calciferol) is named according to the revised rules of the International Union of Pure and Applied Chemists (IUPAC). Because vitamin D is derived from a steroid, the structure retains its numbering from the parent compound cholesterol. Asymmetric centers are designated by using the R, S notation; the configuration of the double bonds are notated E for "entgegen" or trans, and Z for "zuzammen" or cis. Thus the official name of vitamin D_3 is 8,10-seco(5Z, 7E)-5,7,10(19)cholestatriene-3β-ol, and the official name of vitamin D2 is 9,10-seco(5Z,7E)- 5,7,10(19), 22-ergostatetraene-3β-ol (Norman, 2008).

The structures of vitamins D_2 and D_3 and their provitamins are presented in Figure 2. Vitamin D is a structure shown for rings A, B, C, and D with differing side chain structures. The A, B, C, and D ring structure is derived from the cyclopentanoperhydrophenanthrene ring structure for steroids. Technically vitamin D is classified as a seco-steroid. Seco-steroids are those in which one of the rings has been broken; in vitamin D, the 9,10 carbon-carbon bond of ring B is broken, and it is indicating by the inclusion of "9,10-seco" in the official nomenclature (Norman, 2008).

The chief structural prerequisite of a provitamin D is that it be a sterol with a $\Delta^{5,7}$ diene double bound system in ring B shown in Figure 3. The conjugated double bond system in this specific location of the molecule allows the absorption of light quanta at certain wavelengths in the UV range; this can readily be provided in most geographical locations by natural sunlight (or UVB). This initiates a complex series of transformations (partially summarized above in Figure 2) that ultimately results in the appearance of vitamin D_3. Thus, it is important to appreciate that vitamin D_3 can be endogenously produced and that as long as the human has access on a regular basis to sunlight there is no dietary requirement for this vitamin (Ikekawa & Ishizuka, 1993).

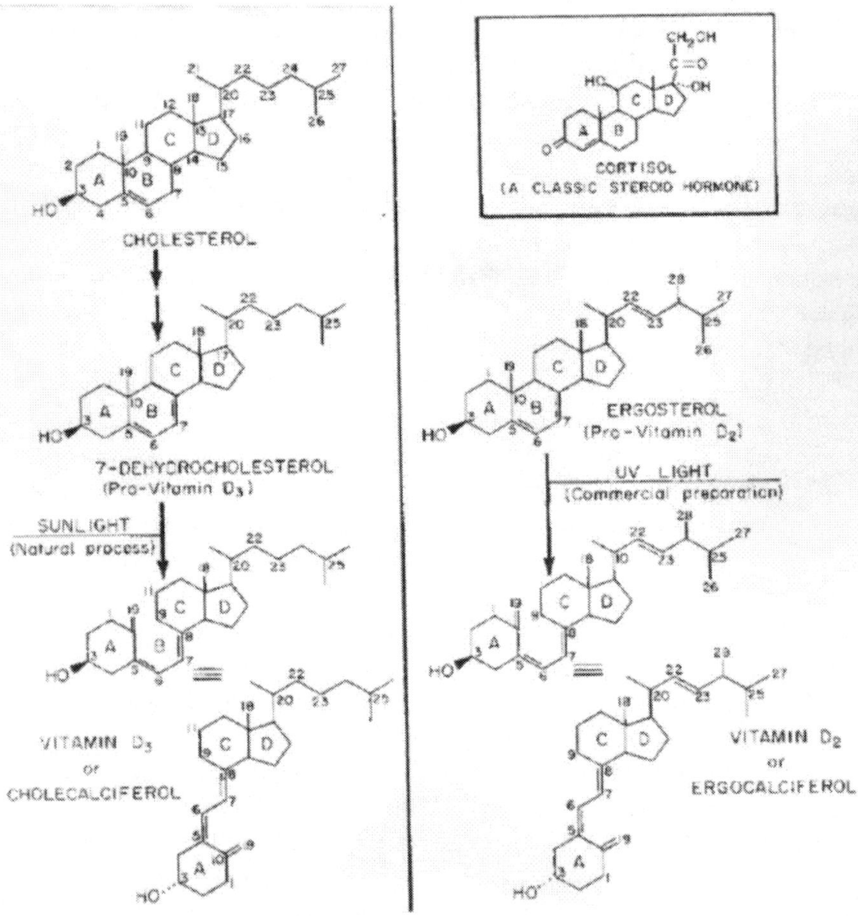

Figure 2. Structural relationship of vitamin D_2 and vitamin D_3 with their respective provitamins, cholesterol, and a classic steroid hormone, cortisol.

Legend. The two structural representations presented at the bottom for both vitamin D_3 and vitamin D_2 are equivalent; these are simply different ways of drawing the same molecule. It is to be emphasized that vitamin D_3 is the naturally occurring form of the vitamin; it is produced from 7-dehydrocholesterol, which is present in the skin, by the action of sunlight. Vitamin D_2 (which is equivalent potent to vitamin D_3 in humans and many mammals, but not in birds) is produced commercially by the irradiation of the plant sterol ergosterol with ultraviolet light.

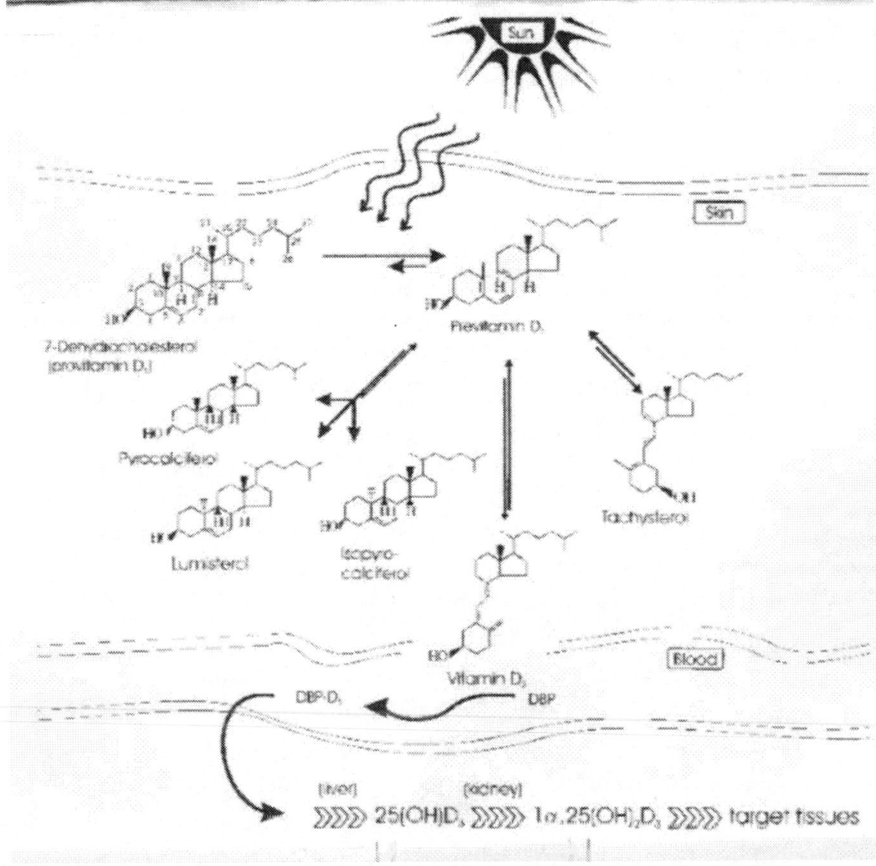

Figure 3. Photochemical pathway of production of vitamin D_3 from 7-dehydrocholesterol.

Legend. The starting point is the irradiation of a provitamin D, which contains the mandatory $\Delta^{5,7}$ conjugated double bonds, in the skin is 7-dehydrocholesterol. After absorption of a quantum of light from sunlight (UVB), the activated molecule can return to the ground state and generate at least six distinct products. The four steroids that do not have a broken 9,10-carbon bond (provitamin D, lumisterol, pyrocalciferol, and isopyrocalciferol) represent the four diastereomers with either an α- or β- orientation of the methyl group on carbon-10 and the hydrogen on carbon-9. The two secosteroid products, previtamin D_3 and vitamin D_3 have differing positions of the three conjugated double bonds. In the skin, the principal product is previtamin D_3, which then undergoes a 1,7-sigmatropic hydrogen transfer from C-19 to C-9, yielding the final vitamin D_3: vitamin D_3 can be drawn as either a 6-s-trans representation or as 6-s-cis representation depending upon the state of rotation about the 6,7-single bond. The resulting vitamin D_3, which is formed in the skin, is removed by binding to the plasma transport protein, the DBP, present in the capillary bed of the dermis. The DBP-D_3 then enters the general circulatory system.

A detailed study of the biochemical mode of action of the fat-soluble vitamin D was not possible until the availability in the 1960s of preparations of high specific activity radioactive vitamin D. As a consequence of efforts in several laboratories a new model emerged to describe the biological mechanism of action of vitamin D_3. This model is based on the concept that, in terms of its structure and mode of action, vitamin D is similar to the classic steroid hormones (e.g. aldosterone, testosterone, estradiol, progesterone, cortisol, and ecodysterone).

The elements of the vitamin D endocrine system include the following:

- in the skin, photoconversion of 7-dehydrocholesterol to vitamin D_3 or dietary intake of vitamin D_3;
- metabolism of vitamin D_3 by the liver to $25(OH)D_3$, which is the major form of vitamin D circulating in the blood compartment;
- conversion by the kidney of $25(OH)D_3$ (functioning as an endocrine gland) to produce the two principal dihydroxylated metabolites, namely $1\alpha,25(OH)_2D_3$ and $24R,25(OH)_2D_3$;
- systemic transport of the dihydroxylated metabolites $1\alpha,25(OH)_2D_3$ and $24R,25(OH)_2D_3$ to distal target organs;
- binding of the dihydroxylated metabolites, particularly $1\alpha,25(OH)_2D_3$, to a nuclear receptor at the target organs followed by the subsequent generation of appropriate biological responses (Norman, 2008).

Over the past 25 years, research efforts have largely focused upon understanding how $1\alpha,25(OH)_2D_3$ generates biological responses. By comparison, the biological actions of $24R,25(OH)_2D_3$ have been relatively less studied. However, evidence has been presented to support the view that the combined presence of both $1\alpha,25(OH)_2D_3$ and $24R,25(OH)_2D_3$ are required to generate the complete spectrum of biological responses attributable to the parent vitamin D (Norman, 1996).

Thus, vitamin D_3 is in reality, a prohormone and is not known to have any intrinsic biological activity itself. It is only after vitamin D_3 is metabolized, first into $25(OH)D_3$ in the liver, and then into $1\alpha,25(OH)D_3$ and $24R,25(OH)_2D_3$ in the kidney, that biologically active molecules are produced (Norman, 1996).

The key kidney enzymes, the $25(OH)D_3$-1-hydroxylase and the $25(OH)D_3$-24-hydroxylase, as well as the liver vitamin D_3-25-hydroxylase, are all known to be cytochrome P-450 mixed-function oxidase. Both of the renal enzymes are localized in mitochondria of the proximal tubules of the kidney. Mixed-function oxidases use molecular oxygen as the oxygen source instead of water. Mithochondrial mixed-function oxidases are composed of three proteins that are integral components of the mitochondrial membrane; they are renal ferrodoxin reductase, renal ferrodoxin, and cytochrome P-450 (Norman, 1996).

The most important point of regulation of the vitamin D endocrine system occurs through the stringent control of the activity of the renal 1-hydroxylase. In this way the production of the hormone $1\alpha,25(OH)_2D_3$ can be modulated according to the calcium and other endocrine needs of the organism. The chief regulatory factors are $1\alpha,25(OH)_2D_3$ itself, parathyroid hormone (PTH), and the serum concentrations of calcium and phosphate. Probably the most important determinant of the 1-hydroxylase is the vitamin D status of the human. When circulating concentrations of $1\alpha,25(OH)_2D_3$ are low, production of $1\alpha,25(OH)_2D_3$ by the kidney is high, and when circulating concentrations of $1\alpha,25(OH)_2D_3$ are high, the output of $1\alpha,25(OH)_2D_3$ by the kidney is sharply reduced (Maiyar & Norman, 1993).

With the discovery of $1,25(OH)_2D_3$ receptors in many classical non-target tissues such as brain, various bone marrow-derived cells, skin, thymus, etc. (Pike, 1991), the view has been expressed that $1,25(OH)_2D_3$ induces fusion and differentiation of macrophages (Kragballe, 1992).

It becomes evident from this method of presentation the role of vitamin D that the nutritionist can focus on the plasma levels of $25(OH)D_3$ and PTH to gain an insight into vitamin D status. Not shown but also important is the endpoint of the physiologic action of vitamin D, namely adequate plasma calcium and phosphate ions, that provide the raw materials for bone mineralization.

2. Vitamin D Deficiency- A World Problem

Although there is no consensus on optimal levels of $25(OH)D_3$ as measured in serum, vitamin D deficiency is defined by most experts as a

$25(OH)D_3$ level of less than 20 ng per millilitre (50 nmol per liter), (Thomas *et al.*, 1998). $25(OH)D_3$ levels are inversely associated with PTH levels until the former reach 30 to 40 ng per millilitre (75 to 100 nmol per liter), at which point PTH levels begin to level off (Holick *et al.*, 2005). Furthermore, intestinal calcium transport increased by 45 to 65% in women when $25(OH)D_3$ levels were increased from an average of 20 to 32 ng per millilitre (50 to 80 nmol per liter), (Gordon *et al.*, 2004). Given such data, a level of $25(OH)D_3$ of 21 to 29 ng per millilitre (52 to 72 nmol per liter) can be considered to indicate a relative insufficiency of vitamin D, and a level of 30 ng per millilitre or greater can be considered to indicate sufficient vitamin D. Vitamin D intoxication is observed when serum levels of $25(OH)D_3$ are greater than 150 ng per millilitre (374 nmol per liter), (Dawson-Hughes *et al.*, 1997).

With the use of such definitions, it has been estimated that 1 billion people worldwide have vitamin D deficiency or insufficiency (Lips *et al.*, 2006). According to several studies, 40 to 100% of US and European elderly men and women still living in the community (not in nursing homes) are deficient in vitamin D. More than 50% of postmenopausal women taking medication for osteoporosis had suboptimal levels of $25(OH)D_3$ below 30 ng per millilitre (75 nmol per liter), (Holick *et al.*, 2005).

Children and young adults are also potentially at high risk for vitamin D deficiency. For example, 52% of Hispanic and black adolescents in a study in Boston (Gordon *et al.*, 2004) and 48% of white preadolescents girls in a study of Maine (Sullivan *et al.*, 2005) had $25(OH)D_3$ levels below 20 ng per millilitre. In other studies, at the end of the winter, 42% of 15- to 49-year old black girls and women throughout the United States had $25(OH)D_3$ levels below 20 ng per millilitre, and 32% of healthy students, physicians, and residents at a Boston hospital were found to be vitamin D deficient, despite drinking a glass of milk and taking a multivitamin daily and eating salmon at least once a week (Tangpricha *et al.*, 2002).

Also at risk were pregnant and lactating women who were thought to be immune to vitamin D deficiency since they took a daily prenatal multivitamin containing 400 IU of vitamin D (70% took a prenatal vitamin, 90% are fish, and 93% drink approximately 2.3 glasses of milk per day) (Hollis & Wagner, 2004); 73% of the women and 80% of their infants were vitamin D-deficient ($25(OH)D_3$ level, < 20 ng per millilitre) at the time of birth (Lee *et al.*, 2007).

However, even in the sunniest areas, vitamin D deficiency is common when most of the skin is shielded from the sun.

3. CAUSES AND EFFECTS OF VITAMIN D DEFICIENCY

Without vitamin D, only 10 to 15% of dietary calcium and about 60% of phosphorus is absorbed. The interaction of $1,25(OH)_2D_3$ with the VDR increases the efficiency of intestinal calcium absorption to 30 to 40% and phosphorus absorption to approximately 80% (Figure 1), (Bischoff-Ferrari *et al.*, 2006).

Conceptually human clinical disorders related to vitamin D can be considered as those arising because of (a) altered availability of vitamin D; (b) altered conversion of vitamin D_3 to $25(OH)D_3$; (c) altered conversion of $25(OH)D_3$ to $1\alpha,25(OH)D_3$ and/or $24R,25(OH)_2D_3$; (d) variations in end organ responsiveness to $1\alpha,25(OH)_2D_3$ or possibly $24R,25(OH)_2D_3$; and (e) other conditions of uncertain relation to vitamin D. Thus, the clinician/nutritionist/biochemist is faced with a problem, in a diagnostic sense, of identify parameters of hypersensitivity, antagonism, or resistance (including genetic aberrations) to vitamin D or one of its metabolites as well as identifying perturbations of metabolism that result in problems in production and/or delivery of the hormonally active form, $1\alpha,25(OH)_2D_3$ (Bischoff-Ferrari *et al.*, 2006; Holick *et al.*, 2005).

Today a lack of the vitamin D has been linked to a host of other maladies, including bone disease, osteoporosis and fracture, muscle weakness, autoimmune diseases, osteoarthritis and diabetes, human immunodeficiency virus, asthma, cardiovascular disease, lung function and wheezing illness, schizophrenia and depression, and cancer among others. How can one vitamin play a role in so many diverse illnesses? The answer seems to lie in the fact that most tissues and cells in the human body (and not just those in the intestine and bone that help fix calcium) have receptors for vitamin D, suggesting that the vitamin is needed for overall optimal health. In addition, some cells carry enzymes for converting the circulating form of vitamin D to the active form, making it available in high concentrations to the tissues locally.

Bone Diseases

In the late 1600s, as people migrated into industrialized cities in northern Europe, their children became afflicted with a crippling bone disease commonly known as rickets. Rickets not only caused growth retardation but, due to the poorly mineralized skeleton, the long bones in the legs became deformed. In addition, vitamin D deficiency caused disruption in chondrocyte maturation at the epiphyseal plates, leading to widening of the ends of the long bones and costochondral junctions. The disease was devastating because the growth retardation and bony deformities were not only disabling, but also childbearing women often had difficulty with birthing because of a flat and deformed pelvis (Holick, 2004).

In 1822 Sniadecki suggested that the reason that children living in the industrialized cities of northern Europe developed rickets was because they were not exposed to sunlight (Sniadecki, 1939). However, by the turn of the twentieth century, >80% of children living in industrialized cities in North America and Europe suffered from this bone-deforming disease. In 1919 Huldschinski reported that children with rickets who were exposed to UV radiation from a mercury arc lamp for 1 h twice a week for 8 weeks had marked radiological improvement of the disease (Huldschinsky, 1919). In 1921 Hess and Unger demonstrated that sunlight could cure rickets when they exposed rachitic children to sunlight on the roof of the New York City hospital and demonstrated radiologically that the rickets had resolved. This led Hess and Weinstock (1924) to investigate independently the use of UV irradiation of food as a way of imparting antirachitic activity (Hess & Weinstock, 1924). Steenbock (1924) appreciated its utility and introduced the concept of irradiating milk as a mean of preventing rickets in children. This led to the fortification of milk with vitamin D, which helped eradicate rickets in the United States and in countries that used this fortification practice (Holick, 2006).

Osteoporosis and Fracture

Approximately 33% of women 60 to 70 years of age and 66% of those 80 years of age or older have osteoporosis (Larsen *et al.*, 2004). Chapuy *et al.* (1992) reported that among 3270 elderly French women given 1200 mg of calcium and 800 IU if vitamin D_3 daily for 3 years, the risk of hip fracture was reduced by 43% and the risk of nonvertebral fracture by 32%. A 58% reduction in nonvertebral fractures was observed in 389 men and women over the age of 65 years who were receiving 700 IU of vitamin D_3 and 500 mg of calcium per day (Dawson-Hughes *et al.*, 1997).

Table 1. Dietary, supplemental, and pharmaceutical sources of vitamins D_2 and D_3.

SOURCE	VITAMIN D CONTENT
Natural Sources	
Salmon	
- fresh, wild (3.5 oz)	About 600-1000 IU* of vitamin D_3
- fresh, farmed (3.5 oz)	About 100-250 IU of vitamin D_3 or D_2
- canned (3.5 oz)	About 300-600 IU of vitamin D_3
Sardines, canned (3.5 oz)	About 300 IU of vitamin D_3
Mackerel, canned (3.5 oz)	About 250 IU of vitamin D_3
Tuna, mcanned (3.6 oz)	About 250 IU of vitamin D_3
Cod liver oil (1 tsp)	About 400-1000 IU of vitamin D_3
Shiitake mushrooms	
- fresh (3.5 oz)	About 100 IU of vitamin D_3
- sun-dried (3.5 oz)	About 1600 IU of vitamin D_3
Egg yolk	About 20 IU of vitamin D_3 or D_2
Exposure to sunlight, UVB radiation (0.5 minimal erythemal dose)**	About 3000 IU of vitamin D_3
Fortified foods	
Fortified milk	About 100 IU/8 oz, usually vitamin D_3
Fortified orange juice	About 100 IU/8 oz vitamin D_3
Infant formulas	About 100 IU/8 oz vitamin D_3
Fortified yogurts	About 100 IU/8 oz, usually vitamin D_3
Fortified butter	About 50 IU/3.5 oz, usually vitamin D_3
Fortified margarine	About 430 IU/3.5 oz, usually vitamin D_3
Fortified cheese	About 100 IU/3 oz, usually vitamin D_3
Fortified breakfast cereals	About 100 IU/8 serving, usually vitamin D_3
Supplements	
Prescription	
- Vitamin D_2 (ergocalciferol)	50,000 IU/capsule
- vitamin D_2 liquid supplements	8000 IU/ml
Over the counter	
- Multivitamin	400 IU vitamin D, D_2 or D_3***
- Vitamin D_3	400, 800, 1000, and 2000 IU

*IU denotes international unit, which equals 25 ng. To convert values from ounces to grams, multiply by 28.3. To convert values from ounces to milliliters, multiply by 29.6;

**About 0.5 minimal erythemal dose of UVB radiation would be absorbed after an average of 5 to 10 minutes of exposure (depending on the time of day, season, latitude, and skin sensitivity) of the arms and legs to direct sunlight;

***When the term used on the product label is vitamin D or calciferol, the product usually contains vitamin D_2; cholecalciferol or vitamin D_3 indicates that the product contains vitamin D_3.

A meta-analysis of seven randomized clinical trials that evaluated the risk of fracture in older persons given 40 IU of vitamin D_3 per day revealed little benefit with respect to the risk of either nonvertebral or hip fractures (pooled relative risk of hip fracture, 1.15; 95% confidence interval (CI), 0.88 to 1.50;

pooled relative risk of nonvertebral fracture, 1.03; 95% CI, 0.86 to 1.24) (Lips *et al.*, 2006). In studies using doses of 700 to 800 IU of vitamin D_3 per day, the relative risk of hip fracture was reduced by 26% (pooled relative risk, 0.74; 95% CI, 0.61 to 0.88), and the relative risk of nonvertebral fracture by 23% (pooled relative risk, 0.77; 95% CI, 0.68 to 0.87) with vitamin D_3 as compared with calcium or placebo (Bischoff-Ferrari *et al.*, 2006). A Women's Health Initiative study that compared the effects of 400 IU of vitamin D_3 plus 1000 mg of calcium per day with placebo in more than 36.000 postmenopausal women confirmed these results, reporting an increased risk of kidney stones but no benefit with respect to the risk of hip fracture. The dietary, supplemental, and pharmaceutical sources of vitamins D_2 and D_3 are presented in Table 1.

The Women's Health Initiative study also showed that serum levels of $25(OH)D_3$ had little effect on the risk of fracture when levels were 26 ng per millilitre (65 nmol per liter) or less. However, women who were most consistent in taking calcium and vitamin D_3 had a 29% reduction in hip fracture (Jackson *et al.*, 2008). Optimal prevention of both nonvertebral and hip fracture occurred only in trials providing 700 to 800 IU of vitamin D_3 per day in patients whose baseline concentration of $25(OH)D_3$ was less than 17 ng per millilitre (42 nmol per liter) and whose mean concentration of $25(OH)D_3$ then rose to approximately 40 ng per milliliter (Jackson *et al.*, 2008).

In one study, evaluation of the exclusive use of calcium or vitamin D_3 showed no antifracture efficacy for patients receiving 800 IU of vitamin D_3 per day (Grant *et al.*, 2005), and some results had an open design in which participants could have been ingesting an adequate amount of calcium and vitamin D separate from the intervention. This called into question the conclusion that vitamin D supplementation had no antifracture benefit (Porthouse *et al.*, 2005).

Muscle Weakness

Vitamin D deficiency also causes muscle weakness (Holick, 2006). Skeletal muscles have a VDR and may require vitamin D for maximum function (Bischoff-Ferrari *et al.*, 2006). A meta-analysis of five randomised clinical trials (with a total of 1237 subjects) revealed that increased vitamin D intake reduced the risk of falls by 22% (pooled corrected odds ratio, 0.78; 95% CI, 0.64 to 0.92) as compared with only calcium or placebo (Bischoff-Ferrari *et al.*, 2006). The same meta-analysis examined the frequency of falls and suggested that 400 IU of vitamin D_3 per day was not effective in preventing falls, whereas 800 IU of vitamin D_3 per day plus calcium reduced the risk of falls (corrected pooled odds ratio, 0.65; 95% CI, 0.4 to 1.0). In a randomized controlled trial conducted over a 5-month period, nursing home residents receiving 800 IU of vitamin D_2 per day plus calcium had a 72% reduction in the risk of falls as compared with the placebo group (adjusted rate ratio, 0.28%, 95% CI, 0.11 to 0.75), (Broe *et al.*, 2007).

Autoimmune Diseases, Osteoarthritis, and Diabetes

Activated T and B lymphocytes, monocytes, and macrophages have a VDR (Mathieu & Andorini, 2002). $1,25(OH)_2D_3$ interacts with its VDR in immune cells and has a variety of effects on regulating lymphocyte function, cytokine production, macrophage activity, and monocyte maturation. Thus, $1,25(OH)_2D_3$ is a potent immunomodulator (Mathieu & Andorini, 2002).

Women who ingested more than 400 IU of vitamin D per day had a 42% reduced risk of developing MS (Munger *et al.*, 2004). Similar observations have been made for rheumatoid arthritis and osteoarthritis (McAlindon *et al.*, 1996).

Several studies suggest that vitamin D supplementation in children reduces the risk of type 1 diabetes. Increasing vitamin D intake during pregnancy reduces the development of islet autoantibodies in offspring (Chiu *et al.*, 2004). For 10,366 children in Finland who were given 2000 IU of vitamin D_3 per day during their first year of life and were followed for 31 years, the risk of type 1 diabetes was reduced by approximately 80% (relative risk, 3.0; 95% CI, 1.0 to 9.0). In another study, vitamin D deficiency increased insulin resistance, decreased insulin production, and was associated with the metabolic syndrome (Cantorna *et al.*, 2004). Another study showed that a combined daily intake of 1200 mg of calcium and 800 IU of vitamin D lowered the risk of type 2 diabetes by 33% (relative risk, 0.67; 95% CI, 0.49 to 0.90) as compared with a daily intake of less than 600 mg of calcium and less than 400 IU of vitamin D (Pittas *et al.*, 2006).

Insight into the important role of vitamin D in the prevention of autoimmune diseases has come from a variety of animal studies. Nonobese diabetic mice that typically develop type I diabetes by 200 days of age reduced their risk of developing this disease by 80% when they received a physiologic dose of $1,25(OH)_2D_3$ daily. Mice that were pretreated with 1,25(OH)2D3 before they were injected with myelin to induce a MS-like disease were immune from it (Cantorna *et al.*, 1996).

These animal model studies have given important insights into the role of 1,25$(OH)_2D_3$ in reducing the risk of developing common autoimmune disease (Manabe *et al.*, 2007).

Human Immunodeficiency Virus (HIV)

Highly active anti-retrovial therapy (HAART) decreases the mortality and improves the quality of life of persons living with HIV infection (Egger *et al.*, 2002). Nevertheless, 17-32% of HIV infected persons living in countries with limited resources experience a temporary worsening of their clinical status after starting HAART despite immunological improvement (Dhasmana *et al.*, 2008). This paradoxical reaction occurs most frequently during the first 3 months after initiation of HAART and is known as immune reconstitution inflammatory syndrome (IRIS) or immune restoration disease (IRD), (Meintjes *et al.*, 2008).

In countries with limited resources, *Mycobacteria tuberculosis* (Mtb) are by far the most common pathogens involved (Colebunders *et al.*, 2006). There is now evidence that vitamin D plays a role in improving anti-tuberculosis (anti-TB) immunity as well as in the regulation of immune responses (Lawn *et al.*, 2005), both of which are crucial steps in the development of IRIS. A double blind randomized controlled trial showed that a single dose of vitamin D significantly enhanced immunity to Mtb among contacts of TB-infected patients (Martineau *et al.*, 2007). Liu *et al.* (2007) showed later that vitamin D acts by increasing the level of the antimicrobial peptide cathelicidin produced by monocytes and macrophages.

Low levels of vitamin D could predispose HIV infected patients with a current or undiagnosed opportunistic infection to IRIS. Indeed, the active form of vitamin D, 1,25$(OH)_2D_3$, has anti-inflammatory activity (Tsoukas *et al.*, 1984) and there is now accumulating evidence for its role in the regulation of human T-cell and antigen-presenting cell (APC) functions (Van Etten & Mathieu, 2005). Furthermore, drug interactions with the enzymatic pathways of vitamin D could favour the development of IRIS (Colenbunders *et al.*, 2006).

The variability in patients' susceptibility in immune dysfunction and thus IRIS could be explained by the polymorphism of the VDR gene known to influence immune cell function, or by polymorphism of hydroxylases regulating the production or the degradation in the bioactive vitamin D (Gupta *et al.*, 2005).

During HAART and immune reconstitution, pathogen-derived antigens are *de novo* recognized by APC, processed and presented to T cells leading to T-cell activation and secretion of macrophage-activating interferon-γ (Baeke *et al.*, 2007). In case of low $25(OH)D_3$ levels prior to HAART, we hypothesize that a defective clearing of pathogens and a delayed negative feedback on macrophage activation due to low $1,25(OH)_2D_3$ production, can lead to excessive granuloma formation and an exacerbated inflammatory response described as IRIS. To avoid macrophage-overstimulation, vitamin D should be given before their massive activation, (e.g. before the initiation of the inflammation).

Our hypothesis could be explored by a case-control study to assess the prevalence of vitamin D deficiency in HIV infected patients on HAART who develop and do not develop IRIS. In cohort studies of patients initiated on HAART, the incidence of IRIS should be compared in patients with low, normal and high baseline vitamin D levels. Moreover, polymorphisms of the VDR, the DBP and the enzymes involved in vitamin D production should be investigated. We also propose to perform functional testing of vitamin D enzymes to find out if an increase of the vitamin D catabolism or a decrease of its production could contribute to low $1,25(OH)_2D_3$ concentrations at the site of inflammation, possibly leading to IRIS.

Asthma

A recent study (Brehm *et al.*, 2009) showed that maternal vitamin D intake during pregnancy has been inversely associated with asthma symptoms in early childhood. However, no study has examined the relationship between measured vitamin D levels and markers of asthma severity in childhood. The relation between $25(OH)D_3$ levels and markers of allergy in asthma severity in a cross-sectional study of 616 Costa Rica children between the ages of 6 and 14 years, was examined. Linear, logistic, and negative binomial regression were used for the univariate and multivariate analysis. Of the 616 children with asthma, 175 (28%) had insufficient levels of vitamin D (<30 ng/ml). These results suggest that vitamin D insufficiency is relatively frequent in an equatorial population of children with asthma. In some particular cases, lower vitamin D levels are associated with increased markers of allergy and asthma severity (Brehm *et al.*, 2009).

Cardiovascular Disease

A growing body of data suggest that low 25(OH)D_3 levels may adversely affect cardiovascular health (Lee *at al.*, 2008). 1,25$(OH)_2D_3$ inhibits rennin synthesis (Li, 2003) increases insulin production (Chiu *et al.*, 2004) and increases myocardial contractility (Zittermann, 2006).

Several mechanisms may explain the link between vitamin D deficiency and cardiovascular disease. First, experimental studies indicate that 1,25$(OH)_2D_3$ participates in the regulation of rennin-angiotensin axis by directly suppressing renin gene expression (Li *et al.*, 2002). Renin overexpression can be produced in wild-type mice by pharmacological inhibition of vitamin D synthesis (Li *et al.*, 2002). Second, vascular smooth muscle cells and endothelial cells express receptors for vitamin D and have the ability to convert circulating 25(OH)D_3 to 1,25$(OH)_2D_3$ (Somjen *et al.*, 2005). Putative vascular effects of vitamin D are wide-ranging and include modulation of smooth muscle cell proliferation, inflammation, and thrombosis (Mitsuhashi *et al.*, 1991). Interestingly, transgenic rats constitutively expressing vitamin 24-hydroxylase, the enzyme that catalyzes the breakdown of 1 to 25(OH)D_3, develop substantial atherosclerosis (Kasuga *et al.*, 2002). Third, vitamin D deficiency triggers secondary hyperparathyroidism. PTH promotes myocyte hypertrophy (Schluter & Piper, 1992) and vascular remodelling (Perkovic *et al.*, 2003).

One study highlights a potential interaction between vitamin D deficiency and hypertension (Wang *et al.*, 2008). Hypertension plays a key role in the development of left ventricular hypertrophy and vascular remodelling. Because vitamin D deficiency may also influence cardiac and vascular remodelling, hypertension could magnify the adverse effects of vitamin D deficiency on the cardiovascular system. Also, experimental and clinical data suggest that vitamin D deficiency directly promotes the development of hypertension (Li *et al.*, 2002) which provides another potential mechanism linking vitamin D deficiency, hypertension, and cardiovascular risk.

On the other hand, Hsia and colleagues (2007) recently reported that use of calcium and vitamin D supplements was not associated with a reduction in cardiovascular events in the Women's Health Initiative. These apparently discrepant findings could be attributable to several factors (Michos & Blumenthal, 2007). First, the Women's Health Initiative was a fracture-prevention trial and was not designed to evaluate cardiovascular risk (Jackson *et al.*, 2008). Second, the dose of vitamin D in the treatment arm (400 IU/d) was far below the amount necessary to correct vitamin D deficiency ($\geq$800

IU/d) or doses used in previous cardiovascular studies (Michos & Blumenthal, 2007). Third, patients in the placebo arm of nearly vitamin D supplements, which resulted in a mean consumption of vitamin D in the placebo arm of nearly 400 IU/d. Lastly, baseline $25(OH)D_3$ levels were not measured in the Women's Health Initiative; thus, the trial did not address whether vitamin D supplementation benefited individuals with vitamin D deficiency, because enrolment was performed irrespective of vitamin D status. It is noteworthy that vitamin D did appear to reduce cardiovascular risk in obese individuals, who are prone to endogenous vitamin D deficiency, and also in those with multiple coronary risk factors (Hsia *et al.*, 2007).

Although the exact mechanism involved in how vitamin D sufficiency protects against cardiovascular heart disease is not fully understood, it is known that $1,25(OH)_2D_3$ is one of the most potent hormones for downregulating the blood pressure hormone rennin in the kidneys (Li *et al.*, 2002).

Thus, there may be a multitude of mechanisms by which vitamin D is cardioprotective. The observation by Teng *et al.* (2003) that renal failure patients who received the $1,15(OH)_2D_3$, were less likely to die of cardiovascular complications helps to support the importance of vitamin D for cardiac health.

Lung Function and Wheezing Illnesses

There was showed that men and women with a $25(OH)D_3$ level above 35 ng per milliliter (87 nmol per liter) had a 176 ml increase in the forced expiratory volume in 1 second. Unsurprisingly, there is significant interest in the children of women living in an inner city who had vitamin D deficiency during pregnancy which are at increased risk for wheezing illness (Black & Scragg, 2005).

Schizophrenia and Depression

Vitamin D deficiency has been linked to an increased incidence of schizophrenia and depression (McGrath *et al.*, 2002). Eyles and colleagues (2005) suggested that maintaining vitamin D sufficiency in utero and during early life to satisfy the VDR transcriptional activity in the brain, may be important for brain development as well as for maintenance of mental function late in life.

Cancer

People living at higher latitudes are at increased risk for Hodgkin's lymphoma as well as other cancers and are more likely to die from these, as compared with people living at lower latitudes (Apperly, 1941). Both prospective and retrospective epidemiologic studies indicate that levels of $25(OH)D_3$ below 20 ng per milliliter are associated with a 30 to 50% increased risk of incident colon, prostate, and breast cancer, along with higher mortality from these cancers (Gorham *et al.*, 2005).

An analysis from the Nurses' Health Study cohort (32,826 subjects) showed that the odds ratios for colorectal cancer were inversely associated with median serum levels of $25(OH)D_3$ (the odds ratio at 16.2 ng per milliliter [40.4 nmol per liter] was 1.0, and the odds ratio at 39.9 ng per milliliter [99.6 nmol per liter] was 0.53). Serum $1{,}25(OH)_2D_3$ levels were not associated with colorectal cancer. A prospective study of vitamin D intake and the risk of colorectal cancer in 1954 men showed a direct relationship (with a relative risk of 1.0 when vitamin D intake was 6 to 94 IU per day and a relative risk of 0.53 when the intake was 233 to 652 IU per day), (Gorham *et al.*, 2005). Participants in the Women's Health Initiative who at base-line had a $25(OH)D_3$ concentration of less than 12 ng per milliliter (30 nmol per liter) had a 253% increase in the risk of colorectal cancer over a follow-up period of 8 years (Holick, 2006).

The relation between sun exposure and melanoma is complicated. Substantial evidence demonstrates that sunlight is an etiologic factor for melanoma, but sunlight also fosters production of vitamin D, which may protect against the disease. A recent review examines these complexities (Egan, 2009). Evidence for vitamin D's protective effect in melanoma comes from both experimental and epidemiological studies. VDRs are present on primary melanomas, and the addition of calciferols to melanoma cells in culture inhibits their proliferation and induces differentiation. Vitamin D production also has immunomodulatory activity; its effects on innate and acquired immunity may play a role in the host defence against melanoma. Moreover, at least two polymorphisms in the VDR have been implicated in melanoma risk. The *f* allele of the *F/f* polymorphism renders the receptor less active; subjects with this allele have a modestly increased melanoma risk. In a second variant, individuals homozygous for the *BAt* allele have higher VDR mRNA levels and reduced melanoma risk. VDR polymorphisms have also been associated with increased aggression and metastases. However, the epidemiological evidence for a protective effect from vitamin D is less consistent. Although one study showed an association between high vitamin D intake and reduced melanoma development, few if any reports have shown an inverse correlation between serum vitamin D levels and melanoma incidence or prognosis (Egan, 2009).

Increased concentrations of $25(OH)D_3$ are used by the prostate cells to make $1,25(OH)_2D_3$, which helps keep prostate cell proliferation in check and therefore decreases the risk of prostate cells becoming malignant (Chen & Holick, 2003).

In an earlier population-based case-control study, Canadian investigators showed that higher vitamin D exposure during adolescence and young adulthood was associated with less risk for breast cancer later in life. Now, these investigators have assessed whether such protection varies by tumor hormone-receptor status. The association between vitamin D and breast cancer incidence was evaluated according to route of vitamin D acquisition (dietary intake or sun exposure) and tumor receptor status (estrogen receptor (ER)-positive/progesterone receptor (PR)-positive [ER+/PR+], 450; ER+/PR-, 110; ER-/PR-, 199). Mean age of cases and controls (1135) was 53; most women were of European descent (Blackmore *et al.*, 2008). Although lower risk associated with vitamin D exposure was shown most consistently for ER+/PR+ tumors, the result might simply reflect that this tumor subtype was the most common. Nonetheless, these findings support vitamin D's beneficial effects on breast cancer risk, regardless of hormone-receptor status (Blackmore *et al.*, 2008).

It has been suggested that if a cell becomes malignant, $1,25(OH)_2D_3$ can induce apoptosis and prevent angiogenesis, thereby reducing the potential for the malignant cell to survive. Once $1,25(OH)_2D_3$ completes these task, it initiates its own destruction by stimulating the CYP24 gene to produce the inactive calcitronic acid. This is a plausible explanation for why increased sun exposure and higher circulating levels of $25(OH)D_3$ are associated with a decreased risk of deadly cancers (Gorham *et al.*, 2005).

There are many causes of vitamin D deficiency, including reduced skin synthesis and absorption of vitamin D and acquired and heritable disorders of vitamin D metabolism and responsiveness (Holick, 1994). Table 2 lists causes and effects of vitamin D deficiency

Table 2. Causes and effects of Vitamin D deficiency (adapted from Holick, 2004; 2006).

CAUSE	EFFECT
Reduced skin synthesis	
Sunscreen use, absorption of UVB radiation by sunscreen	Reduces vitamin D_3 synthesis, SPF 8 by 92.5%, SPF 15 by 99%
Skin pigment, absorption of UVB radiation by melanin	Reduces vitamin D_3 synthesis by as much as 99%
Aging, reduction of 7-dehydrocholesterol in the skin	Reduces vitamin D_3 synthesis by about 75% in a 70-year-old
Season, latitude, and time of day, number of solar UVB photons reaching the earth depending on zenith angle of the sun (the more oblique the angle, the fewer UVB photons reach the earth)	Above about 35 degrees north latitude (Atlanta), little or no vitamin D_3 can be produced from November to February
Patients with skin grafts for burns, marked reduction of 7-dehydrocholesterol in the skin	Decreases the amount of vitamin D_3 the skin can produce
Decreased bioavailability	
Malabsorption, reduction in fat absorption, resulting from cystic fibrosis, celiac disease, Whipple's disease, Crohn's disease, bypass surgery, medications that reduce cholesterol absorption, and other causes	Impairs the body's ability to absorb vitamin D
Obesity, sequestration of vitamin D in body fat*	Reduces availability of vitamin D
Increased catabolism	
Anticonvulsants, glucocorticoids, HAART (AIDS treatment), and antirejection medications binding to the steroid and xenobiotic receptor or the pregnane X receptor	Activates the destruction of $25(OH)D_3$ and $1,25(OH)_2D_3$ to inactivate calcitroic acid
Breast-feeding	
Poor vitamin D content in human milk	Increases infant risk of vitamin D deficiency when breast milk is sole source of nutrition
Decreases synthesis of 25-hydroxyvitamin D	
Liver failure	
Mild-to-moderate dysfunction	Causes malabsorption of vitamin D, but production of $25(OH)D_3$ is possible
Dysfunction of 90% or more	Results in inability to make sufficient $25(OH)D_3$
Increased urinary loss of 25-hydroxyvitamin D	
Nephrotic syndrome, loss of $25(OH)D_3$ bound to DBP in urine	Results in substantial loss of $25(OH)D_3$ to urine
Decreased synthesis of 1,25-dihydroxyvitamin D	
Chronic kidney disease	
Stages 2 and 3 (estimated glomerular filtration rate, 31 to 89 ml/min/1.73 m^2)	
Hyperphosphatemia increases fibroblast growth factor 23, which decreases $25(OH)D_3$-1α-hydroxylase activity	Causes decreased fractional excretion of phosphorus and decreased serum levels of $1,25(OH)_2D_3$

Stages 4 and 5 (estimated glomerular filtration rate <30 ml/min/1.73 m^2)

CAUSE	EFFECT
Heritable disorders- rickets	
Inability to produce adequate amounts of $1,25(OH)_2D_3$	Causes hypocalcemia, secondary hyperparathyroidism, and renal bone disease
Pseudovitamin D deficiency rickets (vitamin D-dependent rickets type 1), mutation of the renal $25(OH)D_3$-1α-hydroxylase gene	Causes reduced or no renal synthesis of $1,25(OH)_2D_3$
Vitamin D resistant rickets (vitamin D-dependent rickets type 2)- mutation of the VDR gene	Causes partial or complete resistance to $1,25(OH)_2D_3$ action, resulting in elevated levels of $1,25(OH)_2D_3$
Vitamin D dependent rickets type 3-overproduction of hormone-responsive-element binding proteins	Prevents the action of $1,25(OH)_2D_3$ in transcription, causing target-cell resistance and elevated levels of $1,25(OH)_2D_3$
Autosomal dominant hypophosphatemic rickets mutation of the gene for fibroblast growth factor 23, preventing or reducing its breakdown	Causes phosphaturia, decreased intestinal absorption of phosphorus, hypophosphatemia, and decreased renal $25(OH)D_3$-1α-hydroxylase activity, resulting in low-normal or low levels of $1,25(OH)_2D_3$
X-linked hypophosphatemic rickets, leading to elevated levels of fibroblast growth factor 23 and other phosphatonins	Causes phosphaturia, decreased intestinal absorption of phosphorus, hypophosphatemia, and decreased renal $25(OH)D_3$-1α-hydroxylase activity, resulting in low-normal or low levels of $1,25(OH)_2D_3$
Acquired disorders	
Tumor induced osteomalacia, tumor secretion of fibroblast growth factor 23 and possibly other phosphatonins	Causes phosphaturia, decreased intestinal absorption of phosphorus, hypophosphatemia, and decreased renal $25(OH)D_3$-1α-hydroxylase activity, resulting in low-normal or low levels of $1,25(OH)_2D_3$
Primary hyperparathyroidism, increase in levels of PTH, causing increased metabolism of $25(OH)D_3$ to $1,25(OH)_2D_3$	Decreases $25(OH)D_3$ levels and increases $1,25(OH)_2D_3$ levels that are high-normal or elevated
Granulomatous disorders, sarcoidosis, tuberculosis, and other conditions, including some lymphomas conversion by macrophages of $25(OH)D_3$ to $1,25(OH)_2D_3$	Decreases $25(OH)D_3$ levels and increases $1,25(OH)_2D_3$ levels
Hyperthyroidism, enhanced metabolism of $25(OH)_2D_3$	Reduces levels of $25(OH)D_3$

*There is an inverse relationship between the body-mass index and $25(OH)D_3$ levels.

Sunscreens are effective at preventing sunburning and skin damage, because they efficiently absorb solar UVB radiation. When used properly, a sunscreen with a sun protection factor (SPF) of 8 reduces the capacity of the skin to produce vitamin D_3 by 95% (Matsuoka *et al.*, 1987). Adults who always wear a sunscreen before going outside are at higher risk for vitamin D deficiency (Matsuoka *et al.*, 1998). Melanin is an extremely effective UVB sunscreen. Thus, African Americans who are heavily pigmented required at least 5 to 10 times longer than whites to produce adequate cholecalciferol in their skin (Holick, 1989).

4. Vitamin D Requirements and Treatment Strategies: Natural Sources and Vitamin D Supplements

Very little vitamin D is naturally present in our food. Oily fish, including salmon, mackerel, and herring; cod-liver oil; and sun-dried mushrooms typically provide 400-500 IU of vitamin D per serving. The major foods that are fortified with vitamin D in the United States include milk, orange juice, cereals, and some breads. Some yogurts and cheeses now are being fortified with vitamin D, whereas other dairy products are not (Holick, 2002). In Europe, most countries forbid the fortification of milk with vitamin D. These countries permit margarine and some cereals to be vitamin D fortified. Our skin is the major source of vitamin D; 90-95% of most people's vitamin D requirement comes from casual sun exposure. An adult Caucasian exposed to sunlight or a (tanning bed) lamp (approx. 32 mJ/cm^2) that emits UVB radiation produces approximatively 1 ng of vitamin D_3/cm^2 of skin. Exposure of the skin to one minimal erythemal dose (a slight pinkness to the skin), raises the blood level of vitamin D_3 to a level comparable to a person taking approx. 10,000-20,000 IU of vitamin D_2. Although aging decreases the amount of 7-dehydrocholesterol on the skin, elders exposed to sunlight are capable of making enough vitamin D_3 to satisfy their needs (Davie & Lawson, 1980).

There are a variety of multivitamin supplements that contain 400 IU of either vitamin D_2 or vitamin D_3. Vitamin D_2 and D_3 supplements are also available in either 400 or 1000 IU capsules or tablets. The recommended adequate intake (AI) of vitamin D for children and adults up to 50 y is 200 IU, whereas the recommended AI for adults 51-70 years and 71+ years is 400 IU and 600 IU (Holick, 1994).

Previously, many studies had established 27 nmol/l as the lower limit (Fraser, 1983). This dietary intake of vitamin D for each population group was rounded to the nearest 50 IU (1.25 μg) and then doubled to cover the needs of all individuals within that group irrespective of sunlight exposure. They termed this amount AI and used it in place of recommended dietary allowance that had been used by US agencies since 1941.

Table 3. Strategies to prevent and treat vitamin D deficiency*

CAUSE OF DEFICIENCY**	PREVENTIVE AND MAINTENANCE MEASURES TO AVOID DEFICIENCY	TREATMENT OF DEFICIENCY
Children		
Breast-feeding without vitamin D supplementation- up to 1 year	400 IU of vitamin D_3/day, sensible sun exposure, 1000-2000 IU of vitamin D_3/day is safe, maintenance dose is 400-1000 IU of vitamin D_3/day	200,000 IU of vitamin D_3 every 3 months, 600,000 IU of vitamin D intramuscularly, repeat in 12 weeks, 1000-2000 IU of vitamin D_2 or vitamin D_3/day, with calcium supplementation
Inadequate sun exposure or supplementation, dark skin- 1 through 18 years	400-1000 IU vitamin D_3/day, sensible sun exposure, 1000-2000 IU of vitamin D_3/day is safe, maintenance dose is 400-1000 IU of vitamin D_3/day	50,000 IU of vitamin D_2 every week for 8 weeks***
Adults		
Inadequate sun exposure or supplementation, decreased 7-dehydrocholesterol in skin because of aging (over 50 years)	800-1000 IU of vitamin D_3/day, 50,000 IU of vitamin D_2 every 2 weeks or every month, sensible sun exposure, or use of tanning bed or other UVB radiation device, up to 10,000 IU of vitamin D_3/day is safe for 5 months, maintenance dose is 50,000 IU every 2 weeks or every month***	50,000 IU of vitamin D_2 every week for 8 weeks; repeat for another 8 weeks if 25(OH)D_3<30 ng/ml***
Pregnant or lactating (fetal utilization, inadequate sun exposure or supplementation)	1000-2000 IU of vitamin D_3/day, 50,000 IU of vitamin D_2 every 2 weeks, up to 4000 IU of vitamin D_3/day is safe for 5 months, maintenance dose is 50,000 IU of vitamin D_2 every 2 or 4 weeks***	50,000 IU of vitamin D_2 every week for 8 weeks; repeat for another 8 weeks if 25(OH)D_3<30 ng/ml***
Malabsorption syndromes (malabsorption of vitamin D_3, inadequate sun exposure or supplementation)	Adequate exposure to sun or UV radiation, 50,000 IU of vitamin D_3 every day, every other day, or every week, up to 10,000 IU of vitamin D_3/day is safe for 5 months, maintenance dose is 50,000 IU of vitamin D_2 every week***	UVB irradiation (taning bed or portable UVB device e.g. portable Sperti lamp; 50,000 IU of vitamin D_2 every day or every other day***
Drugs that activate steroid and xenobiotic receptor, and drugs used in transplantation	50,000 IU of vitamin D_2 every other day or every week, maintenance dose is 50,000 IU of vitamin D_2 every 1,2 or 4 weeks***	50,000 IU of vitamin D_2 every 2 weeks for 8-10 weeks, or every week if 25(OH)D_3<30 ng/ml***

Table 3. (continued)

CAUSE OF DEFICIENCY**	PREVENTIVE AND MAINTENANCE MEASURES TO AVOID DEFICIENCY	TREATMENT OF DEFICIENCY
Obesity	1000-2000 IU of vitamin D_3/day, 50,000 IU of vitamin D_2 every 1 or 2 weeks, maintenance dose is 50,000 IU of vitamin D_2 every 1,2, or 4 weeks***	50,000 IU of vitamin D_2 every week for 8-12 weeks; repeat for another 8-12 weeks if 25(OH)D_3<30ng/ml***
Nephrotic syndrome	1000-2000 IU of vitamin D_3/day, 50,000 IU of vitamin D_2 once or twice/week, maintenance dose is 50,000 IU of vitamin D_2 every 2 or 4 weeks***	50,000 IU of vitamin D_2 twice/week for 8-12 weeks, repeat for another 8-12 weeks if 25(OH)D_3<30 ng/ml***
Chronic kidney disease, Stages 2 and 3	Control serum phosphate, 1000 IU of vitamin D_3/day, 50,000 IU of vitamin D_2 every 2 weeks, maintenance dose is 50,000 IU of vitamin D_3 every 2 or 4 weeks; may also need to treat with an active vitamin D analogue when vitamin D sufficiency is obtained***	50,000 IU of vitamin D_2 once/week for 8 weeks, repeat for another 8 weeks if 25(OH)D_3<30 ng/,l***
Stages 4 and 5	1000 IU of vitamin D_3/day, 50,000 IU of vitamin D_2 every 2 weeks, need to treat with 1,25(OH)$_2D_3$ or active analogue***	0.25-1.0 μg of 1,25(OH)$_2D_3$ by mouth twice a day or one of the following: 1-2 μg of paricalcitriol IV every 3 days, 0.04-0.1 μg/kg IV every other day initially and can increase to 0.24 μg/kg, 2-4 μg by mouth three times/week, or doxecalciferol 10-20 μg by mouth three times/week or 2-6 μg IV three times/week
Primary or tertiary hyperparathyroidism	800-1000 IU of vitamin D_3/day, 50,000 IU of vitamin D_2 every 2 weeks (serum calcium levels will not increase), maintenance dose is 50,000 IU of vitamin D_2 every 2 or 4 weeks***	50,000 IU of vitamin D_2 once a week for 8 weeks; repeat for another 8 weeks if 25(OH)D_3<30ng/ml
Granulomatous disorders and some lymphomas	400 IU of vitamin D_3/day, maintenance dose is 50,000 IU of vitamin D_2/month***	50,000 IU of vitamin D_2 once a week for 4 weeks or every 2 to 4 weeks, need to keep 25(OH)D_3 between 20 and 30 ng/ml (level above 30 ng/ml can result in hypercalciuria and hypercalcemia)***

*These recommendations are based on published literature. IV denotes intravenously to convert the values for 25(OH)D_3 to nanomoles per liter, multiply by 2.486;

**For the specific mechanism of deficiency (see Table 2);

***The goal is to achieve concentrations of 25(OH)D_3 at about 30 to 60 ng per millilitre.

Recommendations from the Institute of Medicine for adequate daily intake of vitamin D are 200 IU for children and adults up to 50 years of age, 400 IU for adults 51 to 70 years of age, and 600 IU for adults 71 years of age or older. However, most experts agree that without adequate sun exposure, children and adults require approximately 800 to 1000 IU per day (Heaney *et al.*, 2003). Table 3 show the strategies to prevent and treat vitamin D deficiency. Since vitamin D_2 is approximately 30% as effective as vitamin D_3 in maintaining serum 25(OH)D_3 levels, up to three times as much vitamin D_2 may be required to maintain sufficient levels. A cost-effective method of correcting vitamin D deficiency and maintaining adequate levels is to give patients a 50,000 IU capsule of vitamin D_2 once a week for 8 weeks, followed by 50,000 IU of vitamin D_2 every 2 to 4 weeks thereafter (Table 3). Alternatively, either 1000 IU of vitamin D_3 per day (available in most pharmacies) or 3000 IU of vitamin D_2 per day is effective (Heaney *et al.*, 2003). Human milk contains little vitamin D (approximately 20 IU per liter), and women who are vitamin D deficient provide even less to their breast-fed infants (Hollis & Wagner, 2004).

The unique problem of estimating total intake of a substance that can be provided in the diet or made in the skin by exposure to sunlight makes it difficult to estimate adequate total intakes of vitamin D for the general population. Accurate food composition data are not available for vitamin D, accentuating the difficulty for estimating dietary intakes.

5. Vitamin D Intoxication

Vitamin D intoxication is extremely rare but can be caused by inadvertent or intentional ingestion of excessively high doses. Doses of more than 50,000 IU per day raise levels of 25(OH)D_3 to more than 150 ng per milliliter (374 nmol per liter) and are associated with hypercalcemia and hyperphosphatemia (Holick, 2006). Doses of 10,000 IU of vitamin D_3 per day for up to 5 months, however, do not cause toxicity. Patients with chronic granulomatous disorders are more sensitive to serum 25(OH)D_3 levels above 30 ng per milliliter because of macrophage production of 1,25$(OH)_2D_3$, which causes hypercalciuria and hypercalcemia. In these patients, however, 25(OH)D_3 levels need to be maintained at approximately 20 to 30 ng per milliliter to prevent vitamin D deficiency and secondary hyperparathyroidism (Table 3) (Villamor, 2006).

The adverse effects of high vitamin D intakes (hypercalciuria and hypercalcemia) do not occur at these new recommended intake levels. In fact, it is worth noting that the recommended intakes for all age groups are still well below the lowest observed adverse effect level of 50 μg/day and have not yet even reached the no observed adverse effect level of 20 μg/day. Outbreaks of idiopathic infantile hypercalcemia in the United Kingdom in the post-World War II era let to the withdrawal of vitamin D fortification from all foods in that country because of concerns that they were due to hypervitaminosis D (Jones, 1990). In retrospect, the vitamin D fortification may have been counter productive because it exposed segments of the UK community to vitamin deficiency and may have discouraged other nations from starting vitamin D fortification programmes. This is all the more cause for concern because hypovitaminosis D is still a problem worldwide, particularly in developing countries at high latitudes and in countries where skin exposure to sunlight is discouraged (Mawer & Davis, 1997).

6. Conclusion and Future Research

Vitamin D deficiency is an unrecognized epidemic in both children and adults throughout the world (Chapuy *et al.*, 1996), even in some of the sunniest climates, including Saudi Arabia and India (Sedrani *et al.*, 1992). The public health consequences of vitamin D deficiency are incalculable. This is especially true for people more prone to vitamin D deficiency, including people of darker skin colour. It is well documented that African Americans are more prone to developing colon, prostate, breast, and a wide variety of others cancers, and that these cancers are much more aggressive compared with the white population. In addition, they are more likely to develop type I diabetes and hypertension, and are at high risk for vitamin D deficiency (Chiu *et al.*, 2004).

Sensible sun exposure in the spring, the summer, and the fall (not during the winter unless one is located below 35^0 north), and education of the public about the beneficial effects of some limited sun exposure to satisfy their body's vitamin D requirements should be implemented (Kennedy *et al.*, 2003).

It has been suggested that exposure to sunlight for usually no more that 5-15 min/d (between 10 AM and 3 PM) on arms and legs or hands, face and arms, during the spring, the summer, and the fall, provides the body with its required 1000 IU of vitamin D. After the limited exposure, this should be followed by the application of a broad spectrum sunscreen with an SPF of at least 15 to prevent damaging effects due to excessive exposure to sunlight and to prevent sun burning. Thus, increasing vitamin D intake from vitamin D fortified foods, and vitamin D supplements, in combination with sensible sun exposure, should maximize a person's vitamin D status to promote good health.

More research needs to be done to know how much vitamin D people need or if can help someone who already has clinical disorders related to vitamin D. Does lack of vitamin D really increase your disease risk? We don't know yet. Scientists and future research will need to look more deeply at the role vitamin D plays in disease prevention and treatment. New research on vitamin and diseases may also lead to the development of new drugs to answer this question.

REFERENCES

[1] Apperly, F.L. (1941). The relation of solar radiation to cancer mortality in North. America, *Cancer Res., 1*, 191-195.

[2] Baeke, F.; Etten, E.V.; Overbergh, L.; Mathieu, C. (2007). Vitamin D_3 and the immune system: maintaining the balance in health and disease. *Nutr.Res.Rev., 20*, 106-118.

[3] Bischoff-Ferrari, H.A.; Giovannucci, E.; Willett, WC.; Dierrich, T.; Dawson-Hughes, B. (2006). Estimation of optimal serum concentrations of 25-hydroxyvitamin D for multiple health outcomes. *Am.J.Clin.Nutr., 84*, 18-28.

[4] Blackmore, K.M. et al. (2008). Vitamin D from dietary intake and sunlight exposure and the risk of hormone-receptor-defined breast cancer. *Am.J.Epidemiol., 168*, 915-918.

[5] Black, P.N.; Scragg, R. (2005). Relationship between serum 25-hydroxyvitamin D and pulmonary function in the Third National Health and Nutrition Examination Survey. *Chesr., 128,* 3792-8.

[6] Brehm, J.M.; Celedon, J.C.; Soto-Quiros, M.E.; Avila, L.; Hunninghake, G.M.; Forno, E.; Laskey, D.; Sylvia, J.S.; Hollis, B.W.; Weiss, S.T.; Litonjua, A.A. (2009). Serum vitamin D levels and markers of severity of childhood asthma in Costa Rica. *AJRCCM, 179,* 765-771.

[7] Broe, K.E.; Chen, T.C.; Weinberg, I.; Bischoff-Ferrari, H.A.; Holick, M.F.; Kiel, D.P. (2007). A higher dose of vitamin D reduces the risk in nursing home residents: a randomized, multiple-dose study. *J.Am.Geriatr.Soc., 55,* 234-9.

[8] Cantorna, M.T.; Zhu Y., Froicu, M.; Wittke, A. (2004). Vitamin D status, 1,25-dihydroxyvitamin D_3, and the immune system. *Am.J.Clin.Nutr., 80(6),* 1717S-1720S.

[9] Cantorna, M.T.; Hayes, C.E.; DeLuca, H.F. (1996). 1,25-Dihydroxyvitamin D_3 reversibly block the progression of relapsing encephalomyelitis, a model of multiple sclerosis. *Proc.Nati.Acad.Sci., 93,* 7861-7864.

[10] Chapuy, M.C.; Arlor, M.E.; Duboeuf, F. et al. (1992). Vitamin D_3 and calcium to prevent hip fractures in eldery women. *N. Engl. J.Med., 327*, 1637-1642.

[11] Chapuy, M.C.; Schott, A.M.; Garnero, P.; Hans, D.; Delmas, P.D.; Meunier, J.; Group E.S. (1996). Healthy elderly French women living at home have secondary hyperparathyroidism and high bone turnover in winter. *J.Clin.Endocrin.Metab., 81*, 1129-1133.

[12] Chen, T.C.; Holick, M.F. (2003). Vitamin D and prostate cancer prevention and treatment. *TrendsEndocrinol.Metab., 14*, 423-430.

[13] Chiu, K.C., Chu, A., Go, V., Saad, M.F. (2004). Hypovitaminosis D is associated with insulin resistance and β cell dysfunction.

[14] *Am.J.Clin.Nutr., 79,* 820-825.

[15] Colebunders, R.; John, L.; Huyst, V.; Kambugu, A.; Scano, F.; Lynen, L. (2006). Tuberculosis immune reconstitution inflammatory syndrome in countries with limited resources. *Int.J.Tuberc.Lung Dis., 10*, 946-953.

[16] Davie, M., Lawson, D.E.M. (1980). Assessment of plasma 25-hydroxyvitamin D response to ultraviolet irradiation over a controlled area in young and elderly subjects. *Clin.Sci., 58*, 235-242.

[17] Dawson-Hughes, B.; Harris, S.S.; Krall, E.A.; Dallal, G.E. (1997). Effect of calcium and vitamin D supplementation on bone density in men and women 65 years of age or older. *N.Engl.J.Med., 337*, 670-6.

[18] Dhasmana, D.J.; Dheda, K.; Ravn, P.; Wilkinson, R.J.; Meintjes, G. (2008). Immune reconstitution inflammatory syndrome in HIV-infected patients receiving antiretroviral therapy: phatogenesis, clinical manifestations and management. *Drugs, 68*, 601-610.

[19] Egan, K. (2009). Vitamin D and melanoma. *Ann.Epidemiol., 19(7),* 455-461.

[20] Egger, M.; May, M.; Chene, G.; Phillips, AN.; Ledergerber, B.; Dabies, F.; et al. (2002). Prognosis of HIV-1-infected patients starting highly active antiretroviral therapy: a collaborative analysis of prospective studies. *Lancet, 360,* 119-129.

[21] Eyles, D.W.; Smith, S.; Kinobe, R.; Hewison, M.; McGrath, J.J. (2005). Distribution of the vitamin D receptor and 1α-hydroxylase in human brain. *J.Chem.Neuroanar., 29.* 21-30.

[22] Fraser, D.R. (1983). The physiological economy of vitamin D. *Lancet, 962-972.*

[23] Gordon, C.M.; DePerer, K.C.; Feldman, H.A.; Grace, E.; Emans, S.J. (2004). Prevalence of vitamin D deficiency among healthy adolescents,.*Arch.Pediatr.Adolesc.Med., 158*, 531-537.

[24] Gorham, E.D.; Garland, C.F.; Garland, F.C.; et al. (2005). Vitamin D and prevention of colorectal cancer. *J.SteroidBiochem.Mol.Biol., 97,* 179-194.

[25] Grant, A.M.; Avenell, A.; Camphell, M.K.; et al. (2005). Oral vitamin D_3 and calcium for secondary prevention of low trauma fractures in elderly people (Randomised Evaluation of Calcium of vitamin D_3 RECORD): a randomised placebo-controlled trial. *Lancer, 365,* 1621-1628.

[26] Gupta, R.P.; He, Y.A.; Patrick, K.S.; Halpert, J.R.; Bell, N.H. (2005). CYP3A4 is a vitamin D-24 and 25-hydroxylase: analysis of structure function by site-directed mutagenesis. *J.Clin.Endocrinol.Metab., 90,* 1210-1219.

[27] Heaney, R.P.; Davies, K.M.; Chen, T.C.; Holick, M.F.; Barger-Lux, M.J. (2003). Human serum 25-hydroxycholevalciferol response in extended oral dosing with cholecalciferol. *Am.J.Clin.Nutr., 77,* 204-210.

[28] Hess, A.F.; Weinstock, M. (1924). Antirachitic properties imparted to inert fluids and to green vegetables by ultraviolet irradiation. *J.Biol.Chem., 62*, 301-313.

[29] Hollis, B.W.; Wagner, C.L. (2004). Assessment of dietary vitamin D requirements during pregnancy and lactation. *Am.J.Clin.Nutr., 79*, 717-726.

[30] Holick, M.F. (2003). Evolution and function of vitamin D. *Recent Results Cancer Res, 164*, 3-28.

[31] Holick, M.F.; Siris, E.S.; Binkley, N.; et al. (2005). Prevalence of vitamin D inadequacy among postmenopausal North American women receiving osteoporosis therapy. *J.Clin.Endocrin.Metab., 90*, 3215-3224.

[32] Holick, M.F. (2004). Vitamin D: importance in prevention of cancers, type 1 diabetes, heart disease, and osteoporosis. *Am.J.Clin.Nutr., 79*, 362-371.

[33] Holick, M.F. (2006). High prevalence of vitamin D inadequacy and implications for health. *MayoClin.Proc., 81*, 353-373.

[34] Holick, M.F. (1994). McCollum award lecture: Vitamin D-new horizons for the 21st century. *Am.J.Clin.Nutr., 60,* 619-630.

[35] Holick, M.F. (1989). *Phylogenetic and evolutionary aspects of vitamin D from phytoplankton to humans, Vertebrate endocrinology fundamentals and biomedical implications,* Pang PKT Schreibman MP ed. Academic Press Orlando.

[36] Holick, M.F.; MacLaughlin, J.A.; Dobbelt, S.H. (1981). Regulation of cutaneous pre-vitamin D_3 photosynthesis in man: skin pigment is not an essential regulator. *Science, 211,* 590-593.

[37] Holick, M.F. (2002). Vitamin D: the underappreciated D-lightful hormone that is important for skeletal and cellular health. *Curr.Opin.Endocrin.Diabetes, 9,* 87-98.

[38] Hsia, J.; Heiss, G.; Ren, H.; Allison, M.; Dolan, N.C.; Greenland, P.; Heckbert, S.R.; Johnson, K.C.; Mnson, J.E.; Sidney, S.; Trevisan, M. (2007). Calcium/vitamin D supplementation and cardiovascular events. *Circulation, 115*, 846-854.

[39] Huldschinsky, K. (1919). Heiling von Rachitis durch Kunstliche Hohensonne. *Deutsche Med.Wochenschr., 45*, 712-713.

[40] Ikekawa, N.; Ishizuka, S. (1993). *Molecular structure and biological activity of vitamin D metabolites and their analogs. In: Molecular structure and biological activity of steroids,* Boca Raton: CRC Press, 293-316.

[41] Jackson, R.D., LaCrois, A.Z.; Gass, M.; et al. (2008). Calcium plus vitamin D supplementation and the risk of fractures. *N.Engl.J.Med., 354*, 669-683.

[42] Jones, K.L. (1990). Williams syndrome: an historical perspective of its evolution, natural history, and etiology. *Am.J.Med.Genet.Suppl., 6*, 89-96.

[43] Kasuga, H.; Hosogane, N.; Matsuoka, K.; Mori I.; Shimakawa, K.; Shinki, T.; Suda, T.; Taketomi S. (2002). Characterization of transgenic rats constitutively expressing vitamin D-24-hydroxylase gene. *Biochem.Biophys.Res.Commun., 297*, 1332-1338.

[44] Kennedy, C.; Bajdik, C.D.; Willemze, R.; De Gruijl, FR.; Bavinck, J.N. (2003). The influence of painful sunburns and lifetime of sun exposure on the risk of actinic keratoses, seborrheic warts, melanocytic nevi, atypical nevi and skin cancer. *J.Invest.Dermatol., 120,* 1087-1093.

[45] Kragballe, K. (1992). Vitamin D analogues in the treatment of psoriasis. *J.Cell.Biochem., 49*, 46-52.

[46] Krause, R.; Buhring, M.; Hopfenmuller, W.; Holick, M.F.; Sharma, A.M. (1998). Ultraviolet B and blood pressure. *Lancet, 352,* 709-10.
[47] Larsen, E.R.; Mosekilde, L.; Foldspang, A. (2004). Vitamin D and calcium supplementation prevents osteoporotic fractures in eldery community dwelling residents: a pragmatic population-based 3 years intervention study. *J.Bone Res., 19*, 370-378.
[48] Lawn, S.D.; Bekker, L.G.; Mille, R.F. (2005). Immune reconstitution disease associated with mycobacterial infections in HIV-infected individuals receiving antiretrovirals. *Lancet, 5*, 361-373.
[49] Lee, J.M.; Smith, J.R.; Philipp, B.L.; Chen, T.C.; Marhiea, J.; Holick, M.F. (2007). Vitamin D deficiency in a healthy group of mothers and newborn infants. *Clin.Pediatr. (Phila), 46,* 42-4.
[50] Li, Y.C. (2003). Vitamin D regulation of the rennin-angiotensin system,.*J.Cell.Biochem., 88*, 327-331.
[51] Li, Y., Kong, J.; Chen, Z.F.; Liu, S.; Cao, L.P. (2002). 1,25-dihydroxyvitamin D_3 is a negative endocrine regulator of the rennin-angiotensin system. *J.Clin.Invest., 110*, 229-238.
[52] Lips, P.; Hosking, D.; Lippuner, K. et al. (2006). The prevalence of vitamin D inadequacy amongst women with osteoporosis: an international epidemiological investigation. *J.Intern.Med., 260*, 245-254.
[53] Liu, P.T.; Stenger, S.; Tang, D.H.; Modlin, R.L. (2007). Cutting edge: vitamin D-mediated human antimicrobial activity against Mycobacterium tuberculosis in dependent on the induction of cathelicin. *J.Immunol., 179*, 2060-2063.
[54] Loomis, W.F. (1870). Although it is still widely regarded as a dietary deficiency disease resulting from a lack of "vitamin D", it results in fact from a lack of sunlight, In smoky cities it was the first air-pollution disease. *Sci.Am., 8*, 77.
[55] Maiyar, A.C.; Norman, A.W. (1993). *Cholecalciferol: physiology. In: Encyclopedia of Food Sciences, Food Technology and Nutrition. ed by Macrae R., Robinson RK., Sadler MJ.,* London: Academic Press, 919-924.
[56] Manabe, Y.C.; Campbell, J.D.; Sydnor, E.; Moore, R.D. (2007). Immune reconstitution syndrome: risk factor and treatment implications,.*J.Acquir.ImmuneDefic.Syndr., 46,* 456-462.
[57] Martineau, A.R.; Wiilkinson, R.J.; Wilkinson, K.A.; Newton, S.M.; Kampmann, B.; Hall, B.M.; et al. (2007). A single dose of vitamin D

enhances immunity to mycobacteria. *Am.J.Respir.Crit.Med., 176*, 208-213.

[58] Mathieu, C.; Andorini, L. (2002). The coming of age of 1,25-dihydroxyvitamin D_3 analogs as immunomodulatory agents. *Trends.Mol.Med., 8,* 174-179.

[59] Matsuoka, L.Y.; Ide, L.; Wortsman, J.; MacLaughlin, J.; Holick, M.F. (1987). Sunscreens suppress cutaneous vitamin D_3 synthesis. *J.Clin.Endocrinol.Metab., 64*, 1165-1168.

[60] Matsuoka, L.Y.; Ide, L.; Wortsman, J.; Hanifan, N.; Holick, M.F. (1998). Chronic sunscreen use decreases circulating concentrations of 25-hydroxyvitamin D: a preliminary study. *Arch.Derm., 124*, 1802-1804.

[61] Mawer, E.B.; Davis, M. (1997). *Vitamin D deficiency, rickets and osteomnalacia, a returning problem worldwide. In: Vitamin D, Chemistry, Biology and Clinical Applications of the steroid hormone.* Norman AW., Bouillon R., Thomasset M. eds., University of California.

[62] McAlindon, T.E.; Felson, D.T.; Zhang, Y. et al. (1996). Relation of dietary intake and serum levels of vitamin D to progression of osteoarthritis of the knee among participants in the Framingham Study. *Ann.Intern.Med., 125*, 353-9.

[63] McGrath, J.; Selren, J.P.; Chant, D. (2002). Long- term trends in sunshine duration and its association with schizophrenia birth rates and age at first registration- data from Australia and the Netherlands. *Schizophr.Res., 54,* 199-212.

[64] Meintjes G.; Lawn S.D.; Scano F.; Maartens G.; French M.A.; Worodria W. et al. (2008). Tuberculosis-associated immune reconstitution inflammatory syndrome: case definitions for use in resource-limited settings. *Lancet Infect. Dis., 8,* 516-523.

[65] Michos, E.D.; Blumenthal, R.S. (2007). Vitamin D supplementation and cardiovascular disease risk. *Circulation, 115,* 827-828.

[66] Mitsuhashi, T.; Morris, R.C. Jr.; Ives H.E. (1991). 1,25-Dihydroxyvitamin D_3 modulates growth of vascular smooth muscle cells. *J.Clin.Invest., 87*, 1889-1895.

[67] Munger, K.L.; Levin, L.I.; Hollis, B.W.; Howard, N.S.; Ascherio, A. (2004). Serum 25-hydroxyvitamin D levels and risk of multiple sclerosis. *Neurology, 62*, 60-65.

[68] Norman, A.W. (1996). *Vitamin D. In: Present knowledge in nutrition (PKN7),* ed. by Ziegler, E.E. and Filer L.J., Washington International Life Sciences Institute, 120-129.

[69] Norman, A.W. (2008). From vitamin D to hormone D: fundamentals of the vitamin D endocrine system essential for good health. *Am.J.Clin., 88*, 4915-4955.

[70] Perkovic, V.; Hewitson, T.D.; Kelynack, K.J.; Martic, M.; Tait, M.G.; Becker, G.J. (2003). Parathyroid hormone has a prosclerotic effect on vascular smooth muscle cells. *Kidney Blood Press.Res., 26*, 27-33.

[71] Phorthouse, J., Cockayne, S., King C et al. (2005). Randomized controlled trial of supplementation with calcium and cholecalciferol (vitamin D_3) for prevention of fractures in primary care. *BMJ, 330*, 1003-1006.

[72] Pike, J.W. (1991), Vitamin D_3 receptors: Structure and function in transcription, *Ann.Revs.Nutr. 11*, 189-216.

[73] Pittas, A.G. (2006). Dawson-Hughes B., Li T., et al., Vitamin D and calcium intake in relation to type 2 diabetes in women. *Diabetes Care, 29*, 650-656.

[74] Schluter, K.D.; Piper, H.M., (1992). Trophic effects of catecholamines and parathyroid hormone on adult ventricular cardiomyocytes. *Am.J.Physiol., 263*, H1739-H1746.

[75] Sedrani, S.H.; Al-Arabi, K.; Abanny, A.; Elidrissy, A. (1992). Vitamin D status of Saudis: IV, Seasonal variations. *Saudi Med.J., 13*, 423-429.

[76] Sniadecki J. (1939). Jerdrzej Sniadecki (1768-1838) on the cure of rickets, cited by W. Mozolowski. *Nature, 143,* 121-124.

[77] Somjen, D.; Weisman, Y.; Kohen, F.; Gayer, B.; Limor, R.; Sharon, O.; Jaccard, N.; Knoll, E.; Stern, N. (2005). 25-Hydroxyvitamin D_3-1α-hydroxylase is expressed in human vascular smooth mucle cells and is upregulated by parathyroid hormone and estrogenic compounds. *Circulation, 111*, 1666-1671.

[78] Steenbock, H. (1924). The induction of growth-prompting and calcifying properties in a ration exposed to light. *Science, 60*, 224-225.

[79] Sullivan, S.S.; Rosen, C.J; Halteman, W.A.; Chen, T.C.; Holick, M.F. (2005). Adolescent girls in Maine at risk for vitamin D insufficiency. *J.Am.Diet.Assoc., 105*, 971-974.

[80] Tangpricha, V.; Pearce, E.N.; Chen, T.C.; Holick, M.F. (2002). Vitamin D insufficiency among free-living healthy young adults. Am.J. Med., 2002, 112: 659-62.

[81] Teng, M.; Wolf, M.; Lowrie, E.; Ofsthun, N.; Lazarus, J.M.; Thadhani, R. (2003). Survival of patients undergoing hemodialysis with paricalcitol of calcitriol therapy. *N.Engl.J.Med., 249*, 446-456.

[82] Thomas, K.K.; Lloyd-Jones, D.M.; Thadhani, R.J. et al. (1998). Hypovitaminosis D in medical inparients. *N.Engl.J.Med.*, *338*, 777-83.
[83] Tsoukas, C.D.; Provvedini, D.M.; Manolagas, S.C. (1984).1,25-dihydroxyvitamin D_3: a novel immunoregulatory hormone. *Science, 224*, 1438-1440.
[84] Van Etten, E.; Mathieu, C. (2005). Immunoregulation by 1,25-dihydroxyvitamin D_3: basic concepts. *J.SteroidBiochem.Mol.Biol., 97*, 93-101.
[85] Villamor, E. (2006). A potential role for vitamin D on HIV infection?. *Nutr.Rev., 64*, 226-233.
[86] Zittermann, A. (2006). Vitamin D and disease prevention with special reference to cardiovascular disease. *Prog.Biophys.Mol.Biol., 92*, 39-48.
[87] Wang, T.J.; Pecina, MJ.; Booth, S.L.; Jacques, P.F.; Ingelsson, E.; Lanier, K.; Bnjamin, E.J.; D'Agostino, R.B.; Wolf, M.; Vasan, R.S. (2008). Vitamin D deficiency and risk of cardiovascular disease. *Circulation, 117*, 503-511

LIST OF ABBREVIATIONS

Vitamin D	calciferol
Vitamin D_2	ergocalciferol
Vitamin D_3	cholecalciferol
$25(OH)D_3$	25-hydroxyvitamin D_3
25-hydroxycholecalciferol	calcifediol
$1,25(OH)_2D_3$	1,25-dihydroxyvitamin D_3
1,25-dihydroxycholecalciferol	calcitriol
UVB	ultraviolet B
AI	adequate intake
VDR	vitamin D receptor
DBP	vitamin D binding protein
MS	multiple sclerosis
PTH	parathyroid hormone
CI	confidence interval
HIV	human immunodeficiency virus
HAART	highly active anti-retrovial therapy
IRIS	inflammatory syndrome
IRD	immune restoration disease
TB	tuberculosis
Mtb	*Mycobacteria tuberculosis*
APC	antigen- presenting cell

ER	estrogen receptor
PR	progesterone receptor
SPF	sun protection factor

In: Vitamin D: Biochemistry, Nutrition ... ISBN: 978-1-61668-273-6
Editor: W. J. Stackhouse, pp. 105-128

Chapter 4

VITAMIN D: BIOCHEMISTRY, NUTRITION AND ROLES (VITAMIN D AND BONE)

Sadaoki Sakai[1, 2], Yoshiteru Miyauchi[1], Yoshiaki Toyama[1] and Takeshi Miyamoto[1]
[1]Keio University School of Medicine,
Shinjuku-ku, Tokyo, Japan
[2]Chugai Phamaceutical Co. Ltd.,
Gotemba, Shizuoka, Japan

ABSTRACT

Vitamin D was identified as a curative treatment for rickets, a human disease causing bone abnormalities. Sunbathing was known to be effective for rickets treatment, and vitamin D was isolated as a factor activated by UV irradiation. Indeed, UV irradiation is required to convert the active form of Vitamin D, 1α, 25-dihydroxyvitamin D3 (1α,25(OH)2D3), from pro-vitamin D. Since 1α,25(OH)2D3 is required to maintain bone and mineral homeostasis, the ingestion of Pro-vitamin D from diet is also important for bone homeostasis. Shorter sunlight exposure or reduced pro-vitamin D intake causes rickets. Basically, 1 α,25(OH)2D3 is synthesized by metabolic conversions in the liver and kidney, and can bind to the vitamin D receptor (VDR) to express biological activities through modulating transcription of target genes. Functional deficiency of the 1 α,25(OH)2D3 metabolic enzyme and the

VDR by gene mutations also results in vitamin D-dependent rickets. 1 α,25(OH)2D3 or its analogs have been used for treatment of renal bone disease and hyperparathyroidism, and later used for osteoporosis treatment as well. Osteoporosis, a disease demonstrating decreased bone mineral density (BMD) and loss of bone strength due to excessive bone resorption, has been treated with 1α,25(OH)2D3 and its cognate analogs. Treatment with active vitamin D3 analogs is reportedly beneficial to correct abnormalities in mineral and bone metabolism in experimental animal models as well as in humans. Administration of active vitamin D analogs in ovariectomized (OVX) animals, a model for postmenopausal osteoporosis, reduces osteoclast number and bone resorption, thereby increasing BMD and bone strength. However, 1 α,25(OH)2D3 induces differentiation of osteoclasts, bone resorbing cells, in a co-culture of osteoclast precursor cells and osteoblastic cells in vitro. Treatment with 1α,25(OH)2D3 upregulates the expression of receptor activator of nuclear factor κ-B ligand (RANKL), an essential transmembrane ligand for osteoclastogenesis, while it downregulates osteoprotegerin (OPG), a decoy receptor of RANKL in osteoblasts, and that stimulates osteoclastogenesis in a coculture system. These discrepancies of in vivo and in vitro data make it difficult to understand the mechanisms underlying vitamin D3 action on bone. Recent advances showed that 1α,25(OH)2D3 directly acts on the osteoclast precursor cells, and downregulates c-Fos protein, an essential transcription factor for osteoclast differentiation, or induces IFN-β, a strong inhibitor of osteoclast differentiation, thereby inhibiting osteoclast differentiation. These findings, at least in part, elucidate the anti-bone resorbing mechanisms of active vitamin D analogs in osteoporotic patients. In this context, the role of Vitamin D on bone metabolism including recent findings is discussed.

INTRODUCTION

Metabolism of Vitamin D_3

In mammals including humans, vitamin D_3 (cholecalciferol) is supplied in two ways, exposure of the skin to sunlight and ingestion in the diet (Figure 1). Ultra violet rays in sunlight induce a photochemical reaction involving 7-dehydrochoresterol, which is synthesized from acetyl-coenzyme A and is a precursor of choresterol, that produces the secosteroid vitamin D_3 in the skin. Additionally, vitamin D_3 can be taken from fish and eggs. Vitamin D_3 must be metabolized by two steps to convert it to its active form, 1α, 25-

dihydroxyvitamin D_3 (1α,25$(OH)_2D_3$, calcitriol) (Figure 1) (DeLuca 2004). The metabolic conversion starts in the liver, where cytochrome P450 25-hydroxylase enzymes add a hydroxyl group on carbon 25 to produce 25-hydroxyvitamin D_3 (Cheng et al. 2003; Ohyama et al. 2004). Vitamin D_3 is transported to the liver as a complex with vitamin D-binding protein (DBP) *via* the bloodstream (Figure 1). Some enzymes reportedly catalyze 25-hydroxylation. In particular, CYP27A1 in mitochondria and CYP2R1 in microsomes are important for appropriate 25-hydroxylation of vitamin D_3 because patients with mutations in genes encoding these enzymes exhibit aberrations in 25-hydroxyvitamin D_3 (25$(OH)D_3$) production (Cheng et al. 2004). Alternate 25-hydroxylation activity by CYP2J3, CYP3A4, CYP2D25, and CYP2C11 are detected in liver microsomes (Ohyama et al. 2004; Shinkyo et al. 2004; Rahmaniyan et al. 2005; Gupta et al. 2005). 25(OH) D_3 also forms a complex with DBP and is transported to the kidney where the second metabolic conversion, 1α-hydroxylation, is performed.

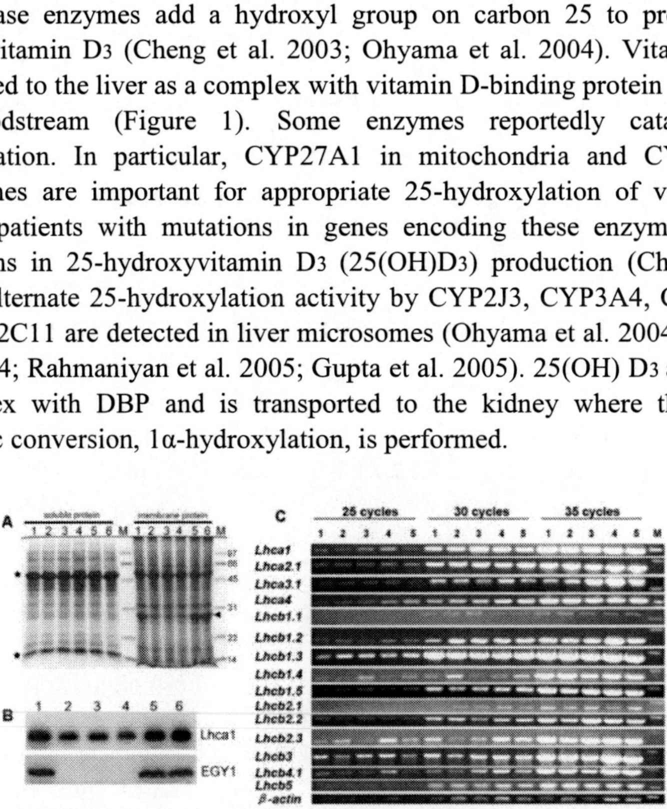

Figure 1. Mechanisms of vitamin D_3 action. Vitamin D_3 is provided by metabolic conversion from the precursor or by ingestion. Metabolic activations of vitamin D_3 are carried out in the liver (25-hydroxylation) followed in the kidney (1 α-hydroxylation). 1 α,25$(OH)_2D_3$, the active form of vitamin D_3, and cognate derivatives circulate as a complex with DBP and are delivered to target organs. 1 α,25$(OH)_2D_3$ activates VDR and induces gene expressions by organization of the transcription factor complex. The products of VDR target genes show diverse biological effects.

The 1 α-hydroxylation of 25(OH) D3 occurs in renal proximal tubular cells, where the responsible enzyme, the mitochondrial cytochrome P450 enzyme 25-hydroxyvitamin D3-1αhydroxylase (CYP27B1), is exclusively localized (Ohyama et al. 2004; Shinki et al. 1997; St-Arnaud et al. 1997; Takeyama et al. 1997). CYP27B1 is the only enzyme that catalyzes the 1 α-hydroxylation of 25(OH)D3, in contrast to the several enzymes involved in

25-hydroxylation of vitamin D3, and is transcriptionally induced by parathyroid hormone in response to a decreasing serum calcium level. 1 α,25(OH)2D3 also forms a complex with DBP, circulates in the bloodstream, and expresses biological activities as described below. Another mitochondrial cytochrome P450 enzyme, CYP24A1, catalyzes the inactivation of vitamin D3. 24-hydroxylation by CYP24A1 increases hydrophilicity and facilitates vitamin D3 excretion out of the body (Ohyama et al. 1989; Ohyama et al. 1991). Since *CYP24A1* is inducible by 1α,25(OH)2D3 signaling and expressed ubiquitously, CYP24A1 is a negative feedback factor that terminates the 1 α,25(OH)2D3 signaling pathway.

Mechanisms of Vitamin D_3 Action

Vitamin D_3 regulates various biological events including calcium homeostasis, immune responses, and cell differentiation (Figure 1). 1 α,25(OH)$_2$D$_3$ action is mediated by the vitamin D receptor (VDR; NR1I1), a member of the nuclear receptor superfamily. Nuclear receptors have the DNA-binding domain (DBD) containing two zinc fingers and the ligand-binding domain (LBD) which includes the transcriptional activating domain, and function as ligand-inducible transcription factors. Therefore, the effects of 1 α,25(OH)$_2$D$_3$ are achieved by regulating the expression of VDR-target genes (Haussler et al. 1998; Norman 2006). Three-dimensional modeling and solutions of the crystal structure of the human VDR LBD and 1 α,25(OH)$_2$D$_3$ show that the 1α-hydroxyl group of 1 α,25(OH)$_2$D$_3$ interacts with serine-237 and arginine-274, that the 25-hydroxyl group comes into contact with histidine-305 and histidine-397, and that the 3β-hydroxyl group is coordinated with serine-278 and tyrosine-143 (Rochel et al. 2000; Yamamoto et al. 2000). This demonstrates that the 1 α-and 25-hydroxylation of vitamin D_3 produce crucial sites for its interaction with the VDR. Some nuclear receptors form homodimers and recognize specific DNA sequences as binding sites, and others heterodimerize with the retinoid X receptor (RXR) to bind to their binding sites. VDR is the latter type and recognizes the vitamin D response element (VDRE), such as direct repeat 3, located in regulatory regions of VDR-target genes. The list of VDR-target genes harboring functional VDRE is growing and includes *CYP24A1* for metabolic inactivation of vitamin D_3, *TRPV6* for calcium absorption, *osteocalcin* for mineralization of the bone matrix, and *p21* for cell cycle arrest at the G1 phase (Chen et al. 1995; Zierold et al. 1994; Meyer et al. 2006; Ozono et al. 1990; Liu et al. 1996). 1 α,25(OH)$_2$D$_3$ potentiates VDR-RXR heterodimerization, changes the conformation of the ligand-binding domain of the VDR, and recruits transcriptional activator complexes to the transcriptional activation domain. The transcriptional activators are the histone acetyltransferase (HAT) and the chromatin remodeling factor, which modulate the structure of the genome by chemically modifying histones and altering chromosome organization so as to facilitate the integration of basal transcriptional machinery including RNA polymerase II. The p160/SRC family forms a complex with the VDR in a ligand-dependent manner and recruits CBP/p300, which produces abundant HAT activity (Tagami et al. 1998). WSTF including nucleosome assembly complex (WINAC) has been biochemically identified as chromatin remodeling factor complex and has bifacial functions; it comes into contact with HAT complex in the presence of ligand and interacts with histone deacetylases (HDAC) complex in the absence of ligand (Kitagawa et al. 2003). The VDR also interacts with vitamin D receptor interacting protein (DRIP) complex, which is also called the mediators complex, without HAT activity and directly bridges to the basal transcriptional complex to induce transcription (Rachez et al. 1998). It is also reported that the VDR directly interacts with the basal transcriptional complex through TFIIA, TFIIB, and TFIID in a ligand-dependent manner (Lemon et al. 1997; Blanco et al. 1995; MacDonald et al. 1995; Jurutka et al. 2000). TFIID consists of the TATA-box-binding protein and associated factors. The VDR associates with the TFIID subunit hTAFII135, and hTAFII135 selectively potentiates VDR-mediated transcription (Mengus et al. 1997). The transcriptional machinery based around the VDR contains regulators for transcription-coupling steps such as NCoA62, which associates with the VDR in a ligand-dependent manner. NCoA62 has been identified as a component of the splicing machinery and may couple VDR-mediated transcription to RNA splicing to ensure appropriate mRNA production (Zhang et al. 2001). Additionally, CAN/Nup214 interacts with the VDR and modulates its transcriptional activity. CAN/Nup214 is a component of nuclear pore complex (NPC), which is built on the nuclear pores that bridge the nucleoplasm and cytoplasm and act as the sole gatekeeper controlling traffic between the two compartments. Since all transcriptional regulators and transcripts move through NPC, CAN/Nup214 may be involved in the localization of the VDR by retaining it around NPC to ensure efficient transcription. It is intriguing that CAN/Nup214 is also known as an oncogene for leukemogenesis, because 1 α,25(OH)$_2$D$_3$-liganded VDR has the opposite activity when inducing the differentiation of some leukemia cells (Miyauchi et al. 2009). In the absence of 1 α,25(OH)$_2$D$_3$, the VDR recruits co-repressor complexes, which produce HDAC activity that blocks the "leaky" expression of target genes. NCoR and SMRT are well-characterized components of co-repressor complexes that associate with nuclear receptors (Nagy et al. 1997). The VDR reportedly interacts with Hairless, a pathogenic gene product for alopecia. Hairless has no structural similarity to NCoR or SMRT, but functions in a similar manner (Hsieh et al. 2003). Other transcription factors come into contact with the VDR and influences to transcriptional activity as a coactivator. For example, Smad3, a signal transducer for TGF-βsignaling, interacts with the VDR in a ligand-dependent manner and stimulates VDR-mediated transcription (Yanagisawa et al. 1999). SRC-1, a member of the p160/SRC family, enhances the complex formation of the VDR and Smad3, suggesting cooperation between these factors. Smad3 may serve as a bridge between the 1 α,25$(OH)_2D_3$ and TGF-βsignaling pathways through physical interaction (Yanagisawa et al. 1999).

The Physiological Roles of 1 A,25$(OH)_2D_3$ and VDR

Vitamin D_3 is closely involved in bone metabolism. Active vitamin D_3 has been used for a long time for the treatment of rickets. It is known that insufficient in sunlight irradiation cause rickets. Rickets is characterized by incomplete bone mineralization, delayed bone growth, and deformation of bone and cartilage. 1 α,25$(OH)_2D_3$ regulates calcium and phosphorous absorption in the intestine and reabsorption in the kidney by binding to the VDR, a member of the nuclear hormone receptor superfamily, to promote bone mineralization by maintaining the blood ion concentration. Therefore, rickets, which is also known as vitamin D deficient rickets, caused by solar radiation shortage causes on active vitamin D_3 deficiency due to a paucity of colecalciferol production. Active vitamin D depletion occurs not only due to a shortage of UV irradiation or malnutrition but also inheritable disorders. The cause of one inheritable disorder is related to defects in the vitamin D_3 activating cascade. Vitamin D-dependent rickets type I (VDDR I) is caused by a mutation in the gene encoding 25-hydroxyvitamin D_3-1α-hydroxylase (CYP27B1), which is indispensable for the production of the active form of vitamin D_3, 1α,25$(OH)_2D_3$ (Kitanaka et al. 1998). *Cyp27b1*-ablated mice show an undetectable 1 α,25$(OH)_2D_3$ level, a high PTH level, and low calcium and phosphorous concentrations in serum, and femurs from these mice show a hypomineralization of the epiphyseal growth plate and thicker osteoid seams (Dardenne et al. 2001). Replacement therapy with 1 α,25$(OH)_2D_3$ administered to *Cyp27b1*-ablated mice cured the rickets and osteomalacia

(Dardenne et al. 2003). Another heritable disease is associated with insufficiency in active vitamin D_3 signal transmission. Vitamin D-dependent rickets type II (VDDR II) is caused by a mutation in the VDR encoding gene (Kristjansson et al. 1993). The *VDR* gene targeted mice exhibit symptoms of VDDR II such as growth retardation, low calcium and phosphorous concentrations in serum, low bone mineral density, infertility, and alopecia (Yoshizawa et al. 1997). VDDR II patients fail to transfer the signal of 1 α,25$(OH)_2D_3$ so that are resistant to active vitamin D replacement therapy. In these ways, active vitamin D_3 regulates skeletal metabolism through binding to the VDR. Since the effects of 1 α,25$(OH)_2D_3$ are mediated by the VDR, the mice deficient for *VDR* are good models for understanding the physiological roles of 1α,25$(OH)_2D_3$. Although VDR knockout mice exhibited the phenotypes resembling the human disease familial 1 α,25$(OH)_2D_3$-resistant rickets the ricketic conditions were rescued by normalization of the circulating calcium and phosphorus levels (Yagishita et al. 2001; Amling et al. 1999). The model mice demonstrated that 1 α,25$(OH)_2D_3$ and the VDR are primarily responsible for calcium and phosphorus homeostasis. To maintain calcium homeostasis, 1α,25$(OH)_2D_3$ induces genes such as *TRPV6*, which encodes the epitherial calcium ion channel, *Calbindin D_{9k}*, which encodes the soluble intracellular calcium transporter, and *PMCA1b*, which encodes the ATPase-driven calcium pump in the small intestine, and then, stimulates calcium uptake (Meyer et al. 2006; Darwish et al. 1992). The mechanism for regulating the phosphorus level is quite different from that for calcium homeostasis. The actions of 1 α,25$(OH)_2D_3$ in phosphorus control are indirect and achieved through fibroblast growth factor 23 (FGF23) (Shimada et al. 2004). Thus, 1α,25$(OH)_2D_3$ organizes mineral regulation *via* diverse pathways. The bone formation involved in mineral homeostasis is believed to be controlled indirectly by 1α,25$(OH)_2D_3$ from observations in VDR knockout mice. On the other hand, *in vitro* studies revealed that osteoblasts lacking the VDR exhibit enhanced differentiation potential, although overexpression of the VDR in mature osteoblasts suggests that it has anabolic effects in bone. It was also reported that the VDR co-operates with Runx2, the master regulator for osteoblastogenesis, in the regulation of bone matrix protein genes in osteoblasts (Paredes et al. 2004; Shen et al. 2005). Additionally, mice that the VDR in their chondrocytes conditionally inactivated have no defects in growth plate development, while the bone of the conditional VDR knockout mice demonstrates impairment of vascular invasion and decreases in osteoclast number (Masuyama et al. 2006). Further *in vitro* analyses clarified that the VDR in chondrocytes directly regulates osteoclast formation through induction of the receptor activator of NF-κB ligand (RANKL) gene, which encodes the essential cytokine for osteoclastogenesis (Masuyama et al. 2006). Extensive work has demonstrated *RANKL* expression is regulated through long-range enhancer and stimulated by 1 α,25$(OH)_2D_3$ and co-operative hormonal signals (Kim et al. 2006). The evidences suggesting the direct effects of 1 α,25$(OH)_2D_3$ on bone formation are accumulated, and led to the creation of a novel pharmaceutical agent that enhances bone mineralization in osteoporotic patients.

1 A,25$(OH)_2D_3$, VDR AND PATHOGENESIS

VDR deficiency is also accompanied by hair loss, alopecia, in humans and mice as well as ricketic phenotypes, while alopecia is not rescued by the normalization of minerals. Conditional inactivation of *RXR*αin skin elicits alopecia indistinguishable from that occurring in VDR knockout mice (Li et al. 2000). In addition, inactivating mutations in *Hairless* encoding nuclear corepressor for transcription factors including VDR results in congenital hair loss in humans and mice (Moraitis et al. 2002; Stoye et al. 1988; Ahmad et al. 1998; Cichon et al. 1998). These findings strongly sugget that VDR, RXRα, and Hairless form a functional complex that controls the hair cycle. Recent reports have suggested that the VDR cooperates with β-catenin, which is the signal transducer of the canonical Wnt pathway, to directly control hair follicle differentiation (Pálmer et al. 2008).

It is interesting that the crosstalk between VDR and Wnt signaling is also involved in tumorigenesis; however, 1 α,25(OH)2D3 is antagonistic to Wnt-induced tumor formation (Pálmer et al. 2001). To date, 1 α,25(OH)2D3 and VDR have been shown to have tumor suppressive effects through induction of cell cycle arrest and differentiation. Some intensive studies have demonstrated that VDR has another anti-tumor effect, the detoxification of secondary bile acids which contain cytotoxic chemicals (Makishima et al. 2002). Primary bile acids synthesized in the liver are important for intestinal absorption of dietary fats and may be the substrate for metabolism by the intestinal microflora to convert to cytotoxic chemicals. It is serious that secondary bile acids injure intestinal cells and result in colon cancer. Two nuclear receptors, farnesoid X receptor (FXR; NR1H4) and pregnane X receptor (PXR; NR1I2), are involved in negative feedback regulation of bile acids in the liver, which represses secondary bile acid production. Interestingly, the intestinal VDR also recognizes some cytotoxic chemicals such as lithocholic acid (LCA) as a ligand and induces the CYP3A genes to detoxify secondary bile acids (Adachi et al. 2005). Treatment with VDR ligands induces Cyp3a11 expression in the intestine and also the liver of PXR-/-mice as well as PXR+/mice, although PXR ligands have no effect. These data demonstrate that the VDR has novel physiological functions that counteract tumorigenesis by sensing and eliminating secondary bile acids.

During metabolic activation of vitamin D_3, endocytosis plays an important role in the kidney. Although the 25(OH) D_3 complexed with DBP had been believed to be absorbed *via* basolateral side of renal proximal tubular cells, megalin deficient mice revealed that the complex is actually taken from the apical side. Megalin is a member of the LDL receptor-related protein family and functions as a multifunctional endocytic receptor. Findings in megalin knockout mice have indicated the critical roles of megalin in brain development and the renal uptake of various filtered proteins including DBP. Deficiency of megalin results in increased urinary excretion of DBP complexed with 25(OH) D_3 and a reduction in serum 25(OH) D_3 levels (Nykjaer et al. 1999). Since the distribution of megalin in the kidney is restricted to the brush-border membrane of renal proximal epitherial cells, it is considered that 25(OH) D_3 is actually filtered by glomeruli and is subsequently reabsorbed in renal tubular cells from the apical side *via* megalin-mediated endocytosis. The intraperitoneal administration of a megalin inhibiting factor reproduces megalin knockout mice phenotypes including the decreased circulating 25(OH)D_3 concentration (Yamagata et al. 2005).

Additionally, recent advances have demonstrated that 1α,25$(OH)_2D_3$ production *via* the controlling *CYP27B1* expression is regulated by FGF23. FGF23 has been identified as the causative factor of tumor-induced osteomalacia and a crucial phosphaturic factor. FGF23 with its co-receptor, Klotho, suppresses renal phosphorus uptake *by* decreasing the mRNA level of *NPT2A*, a phosphate co-transporter in the kidney. Interestingly, it was reported that the regulatory region of *FGF23* contains a functional VDRE and that FGF23 suppresses *CYP27B1* expression to reduce 1α,25$(OH)_2D_3$ level. FGF23 transduces signals through the FGF receptor 1 (FGFR1), but FGF23 alone has no binding activity to FGFR1. Klotho binds to FGFR1, FGFR3, and FGFR4 and creates binding affinity in FGFR1 for FGF23 (Urakawa et al. 2006). Mice deficient in *FGF23* or *Klotho* exhibit similar phenotypes including high serum calcium, phosphorus, and 1 α,25$(OH)_2D_3$ levels (Kuro-o et al. 1997; Shimada et al. 2004). These phenotypes are abrogated by vitamin D-deficient diets in *Klotho* knockout mice and by disruption of *CYP27B1* in mice with a *FGF23*-deficient background, suggesting that the abnormalities in the two knockout mice result from the overproduction of 1 α,25$(OH)_2D_3$ (Tsujikawa et al. 2003; Razzaque et al. 2006). Thus, FGF23 (with Klotho) is the negative feedback factor for 1 α,25$(OH)_2D_3$ synthesis and acts harmoniously with 1 α,25$(OH)_2D_3$ to maintain phosphorus homeostasis. The malfunctions of the megalin-mediated endocytic pathway or the FGF23 and Klotho signaling pathways may be novel pathogenic mechanisms that act through the dysregulation of 1 α,25$(OH)_2D_3$ metabolism.

Active vitamin D_3 regulates calcium and phosphorous homeostasis by controlling the absorption and reabsorption of ions in the intestine and kidney. Parathyroid hormone (PTH) is a endocrine factor that co-ordinately regulates calcium and phosphorous homeostasis with active vitamin D_3. PTH activates CYP27B1 in the kidney and so the production of 1 α,25$(OH)_2D_3$ is strictly controlled by PTH. On the other hand, 1α,25$(OH)_2D_3$ downregulates the mRNA expression of *PTH* in the parathyroid. The main target organs of PTH are the bone and kidney. In bone, PTH enhances the lysis of hydroxyapatite and mobilizes the calcium and phosphorous into the peripheral blood. The serum calcium concentration is monitored by the calcium sensing receptor (CaSR), a 7-transmembrane G protein. The signal from CaSR reduces PTH secretion from the parathyroid and calcium reabsorption in the kidney as a way of regulating PTH and serum calcium homeostasis. In renal failure patients, the serum level of 1 α,25$(OH)_2D_3$ is low due to insufficient CYP27B1 activity in the kidney, and the serum phosphorous concentration is high because of low excretion in urine. In correlation with the decrease in serum 1 α,25$(OH)_2D_3$ concentration, PTH secretion is increased from the parathyroid in order to upregulate CYP27B1 activity in the kidney. However, patients with renal failure can not respond to this signal; and consequently, 1 α,25$(OH)_2D_3$ production is not improved in these patients. A low serum level of 1 α,25$(OH)_2D_3$ and a high serum concentration of phosphorous enhance PTH secretion in the parathyroid; and therefore, these patients exhibit parathyroid hyperplasia. This parathyroid hyperplasia is called secondary hyperparathyroidism (2°HPT) and induces a high concentration of serum PTH and a decrease of bone mineral density (BMD) due to excess mobilization of calcium and phosphorous from hydroxyapatite into the peripheral blood. The administration of active vitamin D_3 analogs is an effective treatment for 2°HPT. The administration of active vitamin D_3 suppresses the excess proliferation of parathyroid cells and PTH secretion, which improves bone homeostasis in renal failure patients (Tsukamoto et al. 2000).

The aberrant responsiveness to 1 α,25$(OH)_2D_3$ results in several diseases. Paget's disease is a chronic highly localized bone disorder that exhibits characteristic bone lesions, which markedly increase osteoclast formation and activity. Although similar numbers of osteoblasts are also present near areas of resorbed bone and the bone matrix in Paget's disease is highly abnormal due to the rapid formation of poor quality bone, it is abundantly clear that osteoclasts are the primary cells involved in the pathogenesis of the disease (Hosking 1981). A striking feature of the osteoclasts from patients with Paget's disease are the large, numerous, and distinctive nuclear inclusions consisting of paracrystalline arrays similar to the nucleocapsids of paramyxoviruses (Rebel et al. 1981). These nuclear inclusions are not present in other bone marrow cells or in non-pathogenic bone tissues in such patients. The basis for the increased osteoclast formation in Paget's disease remains to be elucidated, but it is strongly speculated that a genetic component and nuclear structures are involved in its pathogenicity (Laurin et al. 2002). Osteoclast precursors in Paget's disease patients are hyper-responsive to $1\alpha,25(OH)_2D_3$ and form osteoclasts at concentrations of $1\alpha,25(OH)_2D_3$ that are physiologic rather than phamacogenic. The increased responsivity to $1\alpha,25(OH)_2D_3$ is not due to elevated levels of VDR or to increased affinity of $1\alpha,25(OH)_2D_3$ for VDR. An exploratory study showed that TAF$_{II}$17, a member of the TAFIID transcription complex, is increased in osteoclast precursors from Paget's disease patients compared to those from normal subjects. TAF$_{II}$17 enhances VDR-mediated gene transcription and allows the formation of the transcriptional complex at very low concentrations of $1\alpha,25(OH)_2D_3$. The acceleration of transcription is accompanied by an increase in the expression of transcriptional coactivators for VDR such as CBP/p300 and DRIP205 in osteoclast precursors (Kurihara et al. 2004). These findings strongly suggest that the elevated sensitivity for $1\alpha,25(OH)_2D_3$ in Paget's disease results from increased expression of coactivators of VDR.

BONE METABOLISM AND 1 A,25(OH)$_2$D$_3$

<anti-bone resorptive activity of active vitamin D_3 *in vivo*> It was reported that active vitamin D_3 and its analogs have direct effects on bone metabolism besides indirect effects *via* the control of PTH secretion or promotion of calcium absorption. Maintaining independent living and a high quality of life (QOL) are important clinical issues in an aging society. Bone fractures in osteoporosis patients are one of the major causes of the elderly being bedridden. Active vitamin D_3 analogs have been used in osteoporosis treatment. Osteoporosis is a chronic skeletal disorder characterized by

compromised bone strength and increased risk of fracture (NIH Consensus Development Panel on Osteoporosis Prevention, Diagnosis & Therapy 2001). It is considered that one symptom of senile osteoporosis is the decline of the intestinal calcium absorption. A low serum calcium concentration enhances PTH secretion and accerelates bone resorption in the elderly. Treatments involving active vitamin D_3, 1 α,25$(OH)_2D_3$, and its prodrug 1$\alpha(OH)D_3$ (alfacalcidol) decrease serum PTH and increase calcium absorption (Lau et al. 1999). Thus, active vitamin D_3 administration improves skeletal metabolism and decreases vertebral fractures in osteoporotic patients (Papadimitropoulos et al. 2002). Investigations into the effects of active vitamin D_3 treatment on osteoporosis have been carried out using ovariectomized (OVX) animals, a typical model for postmenopausal osteoporosis.

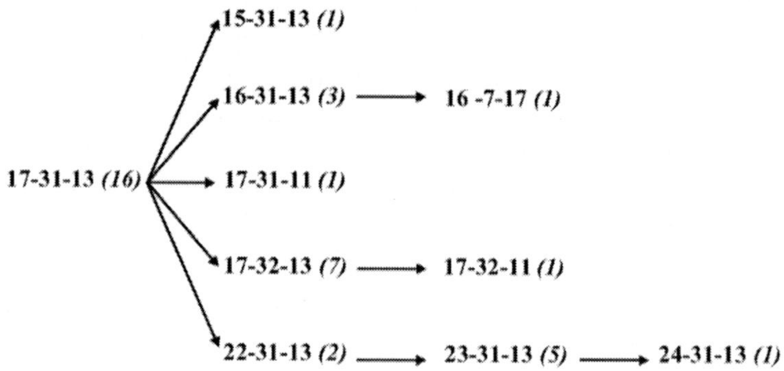

Figure 2. Active vitamin D_3 and its analogs inhibit osteoclast differentiation. Osteoclastogenesis stimulating signal by RANKL is transmitted to transcription factors c-Fos or NFATc1, and upregulates the transcription of osteoclastogenesis stimulating genes. c-Fos also induces IFN-β, a negative feedback molecule of osteoclastogenesis. Binding of IFN-βto IFNAR results in the activation of STAT1. Phosphorylated STAT1 forms ISGF3, a heterotrimeric complex consisting STAT1, STAT2 and IRF-9, and promotes the transcription of the genes containing ISRE domain in the promoter. IFN-βinducible molecules inhibit c-Fos protein translation therby inhibits osteoclast differentiation. In mice, it was reported that active vitamin D_3 and its analogs inhibit c-Fos translation. In human, calcitriol upregulates IFN-βtranscription and inhibits NFATc1 amplification. In this way, active vitamin D_3 and its analogs may inhibit osteoclast differentiation.

It was reported that alfacalcidol administration to OVX rats prevents bone loss but high calcium diet alone does not (Shiraishi et al. 2006). Alfacalcidol also increased bone mass in parathyroidectomized rats that received a continuous infusion of PTH (Shiraishi et al. 1999). This finding suggests that active vitamin D_3 analogs have positive effects on bone metabolism besides regulating PTH secretion and calcium absorption. OVX animals shows high bone turnover characterized by excess bone resorption and bone formation. High bone turnover results in immature bone mineralization, which decreases BMD and bone strength. The increased bone resorption occurs through the activation of osteoclast differentiation and acceleration of bone resorption. Treatment of OVX rats with alfacalcidol reduces bone resorption without a significant elevation of serum calcium (Shiraishi et al. 2000) and decreases the pool of osteoclast precursor cells in bone marrow (Shibata et al. 2002). Thus, the evidence for an *in vivo* anti-osteoclastic effect of active vitamin D_3 is accumulating.

<Active vitamin D_3 action in osteoclastogenesis *in vitro*> Nevertheless, despite its anti-bone resorbing effects in vivo, active vitamin D3 is considered to be a bone resorbing hormone. Bone homeostasis is controlled via the balance of bone formation by osteoblasts and bone resorption by osteoclasts. Osteoblasts are differentiated from stromal cells, and osteoclasts are differentiated from hematopoietic cells. Osteoblasts express receptor activator of nuclear factor k-B ligand (RANKL) and osteoprotegerin (OPG), a decoy receptor of RANKL, and play a crucial role in osteoclast differentiation. RANKL is an essential transmembrane ligand for osteoclastogenesis, and OPG inhibits its signaling. Active vitamin D3 binds to VDR on osteoblasts and upregulates RANKL expression and consequently enhances osteoclastogenesis in in vitro cocultures of osteoblasts and osteoclast precursor cells (Suda et al. 1999). The discrepancy in the effects of active vitamin D3 between its anti-bone resorbing effect in vivo and the osteoclastogenesis supporting effect in vitro has been investigated. Active vitamin D3 inhibits osteoclastogenesis by promoting the signal transduction of RANKL. When RANKL binds to RANK, a receptor for RANKL, on osteoclast precursor cells, the transcription factor c-Fos is upregulated. c-Fos is indispensable for osteoclastogenesis, and c-fos-ablated mice have no osteoclasts and exhibit osteopetrosis. c-Fos upregulates the transcription of NFATc1, a transcription factor that integrates RANKL signaling (Takayanagi et al. 2002). c-Fos also induces the transcription of interferon beta (IFN-β),which regulates the negative feedback of RANKL. Osteoclast precursor cells in bone marrow differentiate to osteoclasts under stimulation from macrophage colony stimulating factor (M-CSF) and RANKL in vitro without osteoblastic cells. This monoculture system was used to elucidate the direct effects of active vitamin D3 on osteoclast precursor cells in osteoclastogenesis. In mouse bone marrow, 1 α,25(OH)2D3 and its analogs act directly on osteoclast precursor cells and inhibit c-Fos translation (Figure 2)

(Takasu et al. 2006). In human bone marrow osteoclast precursor cells, 1 α,25(OH)2D3 also inhibits osteoclastogenesis by inducing IFN-β expression (Figure 2) (Sakai et al. 2009). In anti-osteoclastogenesis in vitro above mentioned, the required dose of 1 α,25(OH)2D3 is 1-10 nM. The physiological serum concentration of 1 α,25(OH)2D3 has been reported to be approximately 0.1 nM; however, the administration of 1 α,25(OH)2D3 or its analogs such as alfacalcidol was reported to increase the local concentration of 1 α,25(OH)2D3 in bone (Kitanaka et al. 1998; Koike et al. 1998). These findings partially elucidate the mechanisms of the anti-osteoclastogenic effects of active vitamin D3.

FUTURE DIRECTIONS

In contrast to the central pathway for 1 α,25(OH)$_2$D$_3$ production, the local synthesis of 1α,25(OH)$_2$D$_3$ has been investigated. Recently, *CYP27B1* and *VDR* expression were found to be activated in macrophages stimulated by the Toll-like receptor (TLR) (Liu et al. 2006). This unexpected result indicates that the effect of 1 α,25(OH)$_2$D$_3$ is a target of the innate immune response and led to the identification of a novel target gene of VDR, cathelicidin, an anti-microbial peptide that is involved in counteracting microbial infections downstream of TLR. The regulatory region of the *cathelicidin* gene contains the functional VDRE, and treatment with 1 α,25(OH)$_2$D$_3$ induces expression of the *cathelicidin* in macrophages, monocytes, neutrophils and keratinocytes (Gombart et al. 2005). These findings suggest that 1 α,25(OH)$_2$D$_3$ plays a novel physiological role in innate immunity, and furthermore, that extra-renal 1 α,25(OH)$_2$D$_3$ production has physiological relevance.

Since alfacalcidol became available for the treatment of vitamin D metabolic abnormalities, the application of active vitamin D analogs to other diseases has been tested. 22-oxacalcitriol (Brown et al. 1989) and 19-nor-1,25(OH)$_2$D$_2$ which have short serum half-lives, are used for 2°HPT treatment as a way of inhibiting PTH production and secretion. Analogs that have anti-proliferative effects on keratinocyte such as 22-oxacalcitriol (Morimoto et al. 1989) or calcipotriol are used for psoriasis. These analogs successfully isolated the calcemic effect from the main action for treatment. ED-71, a new active vitamin D$_3$ analog, is under clinical development for the treatment of osteoporosis. ED-71 has a stronger inhibitory effect on bone resorption than alfacalcidol in OVX rats (Uchiyama et al. 2002) and increases bone mass in osteoporotic patients under vitamin D supplementation (Matsumoto et al. 2005). It was reported that active vitamin D$_3$ inhibits the early stage of osteoclast differentiation during high bone turnover such as that seen in osteoporosis. These reports suggest that active vitamin D_3 therapy reduces the number of osteoclast precursor cells. Recently, it was identified the osteoclast precursor pool, the cell cycle – arrested quiescent osteoclast precursors (QuOP), which readily differentiate into osteoclast without cell division (Mizoguchi et al. 2009). QuOP respond to RANKL signaling and differentiate into mature osteoclast within three days. In osteoporosis patients and OVX animals, osteoclasts are differentiated from QuOP. The chronic acceleration of osteoclastogenesis may cause a depletion of QuOP and so the supply of QuOP will be increased. It is understandable that the inhibitory effect of active vitamin D_3 on osteoclastogenesis in osteoporotic patients and OVX animals is due to the inhibition of QuOP supply. Further studies are needed to elucidate the anti osteoporotic mechanisms of active vitamin D_3; however, the finding of the direct inhibitory effect of active vitamin D_3 on osteoclast differentiation may aid the development of osteoporosis therapies.

Conclusion

Numerous studies have elucidated the metabolism of vitamin D_3, mechanism of its actions, the pathogenicity and the pharmacological applications. The vitamin D_3 has the novel activities for the regulation of immune systems in addition to the regulatory roles for mineral homeostasis and tumor suppression. Therefore, it is strongly expected the potency of vitamin D_3 for diverse pharmacological development.

References

Adachi R, Honma Y, Masuno H, Kawana K, Shimomura I, Yamada S, Makishima M. (2005). Selective activation of vitamin D receptor by lithocholic acid acetate, a bile acid derivative. *J Lipid Res.*, 46, 46-57.

Ahmad W, Faiyaz ul Haque M, Brancolini V, Tsou HC, ul Haque S, Lam H, Aita VM, Owen J, deBlaquiere M, Frank J, Cserhalmi-Friedman PB, Leask A, McGrath JA, Peacocke M, Ahmad M, Ott J, Christiano AM. (1998). Alopecia universalis associated with a mutation in the human hairless gene. *Science*, 279, 720-4.

Amling M, Priemel M, Holzmann T, Chapin K, Rueger JM, Baron R, Demay MB. (1999). Rescue of the skeletal phenotype of vitamin D receptor-ablated mice in the setting of normal mineral ion homeostasis: formal histomorphometric and biomechanical analyses. *Endocrinology*, 140, 4982-7.

Blanco JC, Wang IM, Tsai SY, Tsai MJ, O'Malley BW, Jurutka PW, Haussler MR, Ozato K. (1995). *Transcription factor TFIIB and the vitamin D receptor cooperatively activate ligand-dependent transcription.* Proc Natl Acad Sci U S A., 92, 1535-9.

Brown AJ, Ritter CR, Finch JL, Morrissey J, Martin KJ, Murayama E, Nishii Y, Slatopolsky E. (1989). The noncalcemic analogue of vitamin D, 22-oxacalcitriol, suppresses parathyroid hormone synthesis and secretion. *J Clin Invest.*, 84, 728-32.

Chen KS, DeLuca HF. (1995). Cloning of the human 1 alpha,25-dihydroxyvitamin D-3 24-hydroxylase gene promoter and identification of two vitamin D-responsive elements. *Biochim Biophys Acta.*, 1263, 1-9.

Cheng JB, Levine MA, Bell NH, Mangelsdorf DJ, Russell DW. (2004). *Genetic evidence that the human CYP2R1 enzyme is a key vitamin D 25-hydroxylase.* Proc Natl Acad Sci U S A., 101, 7711-5.

Cheng JB, Motola DL, Mangelsdorf DJ, Russell DW. (2003). De-orphanization of cytochrome P450 2R1: a microsomal vitamin D 25-hydroxilase. *J Biol Chem.*, 278, 38084-93.

Cichon S, Anker M, Vogt IR, Rohleder H, Pützstück M, Hillmer A, Farooq SA, Al-Dhafri KS, Ahmad M, Haque S, Rietschel M, Propping P, Kruse R, Nöthen MM. (1998). Cloning, genomic organization, alternative transcripts and mutational analysis of the gene responsible for autosomal recessive universal congenital alopecia. *Hum Mol Genet.*, 7, 1671-9.

Dardenne O, Prud'homme J, Arabian A, Glorieux FH, St-Arnaud R. (2001). Targeted inactivation of the 25-hydroxyvitamin D(3)-1(alpha)-hydroxylase gene (CYP27B1) creates an animal model of pseudovitamin D-deficiency rickets. *Endocrinology*, 142, 3135-41.

Dardenne O, Prudhomme J, Hacking SA, Glorieux FH, St-Arnaud R. (2003). Rescue of the pseudo-vitamin D deficiency rickets phenotype of CYP27B1-deficient mice by treatment with 1,25-dihydroxyvitamin D3: biochemical, histomorphometric, and biomechanical analyses. *J Bone Miner Res.*, 18, 637-43.

Darwish HM, DeLuca HF. (1992). *Identification of a 1,25-dihydroxyvitamin D3-response element in the 5'-flanking region of the rat calbindin D-9k gene.* Proc Natl Acad Sci U S A., 89, 603-7.

DeLuca HF. (2004). Overview of general physiologic features and functions of vitamin D. Am *J Clin Nutr.*, 80(6 Suppl), 1689S-96S.

Gombart AF, Borregaard N, Koeffler HP. (2005). Human cathelicidin antimicrobial peptide (CAMP) gene is a direct target of the vitamin D receptor and is strongly up-regulated in myeloid cells by 1,25-dihydroxyvitamin D3. *FASEB J.*, 19, 1067-77.

Gupta RP, He YA, Patrick KS, Halpert JR, Bell NH. (2005). CYP3A4 is a vitamin D-24-and 25-hydroxylase: analysis of structure function by site-directed mutagenesis. *J Clin Endocrinol Metab.*, 90, 1210-9.

Haussler MR, Whitfield GK, Haussler CA, Hsieh JC, Thompson PD, Selznick SH, Dominguez CE, Jurutka PW. (1998). The nuclear vitamin D receptor: biological and molecular regulatory properties revealed. *J Bone Miner Res.*, 13, 325-49.

Hosking DJ. (1981). Paget's disease of bone. *Br Med J* (Clin Res Ed)., 283, 686-8.

Hsieh JC, Sisk JM, Jurutka PW, Haussler CA, Slater SA, Haussler MR, Thompson CC. (2003). Physical and functional interaction between the vitamin D receptor and hairless corepressor, two proteins required for hair cycling. *J Biol Chem.*, 278, 38665-74.

Jurutka PW, Remus LS, Whitfield GK, Thompson PD, Hsieh JC, Zitzer H, Tavakkoli P, Galligan MA, Dang HT, Haussler CA, Haussler MR. (2000). The polymorphic N terminus in human vitamin D receptor isoforms influences transcriptional activity by modulating interaction with transcription factor IIB. *Mol Endocrinol.*, 14, 401-20.

Kim S, Yamazaki M, Zella LA, Shevde NK, Pike JW. (2006). Activation of receptor activator of NF-kappaB ligand gene expression by 1,25-dihydroxyvitamin D3 is mediated through multiple long-range enhancers. *Mol Cell Biol.,* 26, 6469-86.

Kitagawa H, Fujiki R, Yoshimura K, Mezaki Y, Uematsu Y, Matsui D, Ogawa S, Unno K, Okubo M, Tokita A, Nakagawa T, Ito T, Ishimi Y, Nagasawa H, Matsumoto T, Yanagisawa J, Kato S. (2003). The chromatin-remodeling complex WINAC targets a nuclear receptor to promoters and is impaired in Williams syndrome. *Cell,* 113, 905-17.

Kitanaka S, Takeyama K, Murayama A, Sato T, Okumura K, Nogami M, Hasegawa Y, Niimi H, Yanagisawa J, Tanaka T, Kato S. (1998). Inactivating mutations in the 25-hydroxyvitamin D3 1alpha-hydroxylase gene in patients with pseudovitamin D-deficiency rickets. *N Engl J Med.,* 338, 653-61.

Koike N, Ichikawa F, Nishii Y, Stumpf WE. (1998). Sustained osteoblast nuclear receptor binding of converted 1alpha, 25-dihydroxyvitamin D3 after administration of 3H-1alpha-hydroxyvitamin D3: a combined receptor autoradiography and radioassay time course study with comparison to 3H-1alpha, 25-dihydroxyvitamin D3. *Calcif Tissue Int.*, 63, 391-5.

Kristjansson K, Rut AR, Hewison M, O'Riordan JL, Hughes MR. (1993). Two mutations in the hormone binding domain of the vitamin D receptor cause tissue resistance to 1,25 dihydroxyvitamin D3. *J Clin Invest.*, 92, 12-6.

Kurihara N, Ishizuka S, Demulder A, Menaa C, Roodman GD. (2004). Paget's disease-a VDR coactivator disease? *J Steroid Biochem Mol Biol.*, 89-90 321-5.

Kuro-o M, Matsumura Y, Aizawa H, Kawaguchi H, Suga T, Utsugi T, Ohyama Y, Kurabayashi M, Kaname T, Kume E, Iwasaki H, Iida A, Shiraki-Iida T, Nishikawa S, Nagai R, Nabeshima YI. (1997). Mutation of the mouse klotho gene leads to a syndrome resembling ageing. *Nature*, 390, 45-51.

Lau KH, Baylink DJ. (1999). Vitamin D therapy of osteoporosis: plain vitamin D therapy versus active vitamin D analog (D-hormone) therapy. *Calcif Tissue Int.*, 65, 295-306.

Laurin N, Brown JP, Morissette J, Raymond V. (2002). Recurrent mutation of the gene encoding sequestosome 1 (SQSTM1/p62) in Paget disease of bone. *Am J Hum Genet.*, 70, 1582-8.

Lemon BD, Fondell JD, Freedman LP. (1997). Retinoid X receptor:vitamin D3 receptor heterodimers promote stable preinitiation complex formation and direct 1,25-dihydroxyvitamin D3-dependent cell-free transcription. *Mol Cell Biol.*, 17, 1923-37.

Li M, Indra AK, Warot X, Brocard J, Messaddeq N, Kato S, Metzger D, Chambon P. (2000). Skin abnormalities generated by temporally controlled RXRalpha mutations in mouse epidermis. *Nature*, 407, 633-6.

Liu M, Lee MH, Cohen M, Bommakanti M, Freedman LP. (1996). Transcriptional activation of the Cdk inhibitor p21 by vitamin D3 leads to the induced differentiation of the myelomonocytic cell line U937. *Genes Dev.*, 10, 142-53.

Liu PT, Stenger S, Li H, Wenzel L, Tan BH, Krutzik SR, Ochoa MT, Schauber J, Wu K, Meinken C, Kamen DL, Wagner M, Bals R, Steinmeyer A, Zügel U, Gallo RL, Eisenberg D, Hewison M, Hollis BW, Adams JS, Bloom BR, Modlin RL. (2006). Toll-like receptor triggering of a vitamin D-mediated human antimicrobial response. *Science*, 311, 1770-3.

MacDonald PN, Sherman DR, Dowd DR, Jefcoat SC Jr, DeLisle RK. (1995). The vitamin D receptor interacts with general transcription factor IIB. *J Biol Chem.*, 270, 4748-52.

Makishima M, Lu TT, Xie W, Whitfield GK, Domoto H, Evans RM, Haussler MR, Mangelsdorf DJ. (2002). Vitamin D receptor as an intestinal bile acid sensor. *Science*. 296, 1313-6.

Masuyama R, Stockmans I, Torrekens S, Van Looveren R, Maes C, Carmeliet P, Bouillon R, Carmeliet G. (2006). Vitamin D receptor in chondrocytes promotes osteoclastogenesis and regulates FGF23 production in osteoblasts. *J Clin Invest.*, 116, 3150-9.

Matsumoto T, Miki T, Hagino H, Sugimoto T, Okamoto S, Hirota T, Tanigawara Y, Hayashi Y, Fukunaga M, Shiraki M, Nakamura T. (2005). A new active vitamin D, ED-71, increases bone mass in osteoporotic patients under vitamin D supplementation: a randomized, double-blind, placebo-controlled clinical trial. *J Clin Endocrinol Metab.*, 90, 5031-6.

Mengus G, May M, Carré L, Chambon P, Davidson I. (1997). Human TAF(II)135 potentiates transcriptional activation by the AF-2s of the retinoic acid, vitamin D3, and thyroid hormone receptors in mammalian cells. *Genes Dev.,* 11, 1381-95.

Meyer MB, Watanuki M, Kim S, Shevde NK, Pike JW. (2006). The human transient receptor potential vanilloid type 6 distal promoter contains multiple vitamin D receptor binding sites that mediate activation by 1,25-dihydroxyvitamin D3 in intestinal cells. *Mol Endocrinol.*, 20, 1447-61.

Miyauchi Y, Sakaguchi N, Okada T, Makishima M, Ozono K, Michigami T. (2009). Oncogenic nucleoporin CAN/Nup214 interacts with vitamin D receptor and modulates its function. *J Cell Biochem.,* 106, 1090-101

Mizoguchi T, Muto A, Udagawa N, Arai A, Yamashita T, Hosoya A, Ninomiya T, Nakamura H, Yamamoto Y, Kinugawa S, Nakamura M, Nakamichi Y, Kobayashi Y, Nagasawa S, Oda K, Tanaka H, Tagaya M, Penninger JM, Ito M, Takahashi N. (2009). Identification of cell cycle-arrested quiescent osteoclast precursors in vivo. *J Cell Biol.*,184, 541-54.

Moraitis AN, Giguère V, Thompson CC. (2002). Novel mechanism of nuclear receptor corepressor interaction dictated by activation function 2 helix determinants. *Mol Cell Biol.,* 22, 6831-41.

Morimoto S, Imanaka S, Koh E, Shiraishi T, Nabata T, Kitano S, Miyashita Y, Nishii Y, Ogihara T. (1989). Comparison of the inhibitions of proliferation of normal and psoriatic fibroblasts by 1 alpha,25-dihydroxyvitamin D3 and synthetic analogues of vitamin D3 with an oxygen atom in their side chain. *Biochem Int.*, 19, 1143-9.

Nagy L, Kao HY, Chakravarti D, Lin RJ, Hassig CA, Ayer DE, Schreiber SL, Evans RM. (1997). Nuclear receptor repression mediated by a complex containing SMRT, mSin3A, and histone deacetylase. *Cell*, 89. 373-80.

NIH Consensus Development Panel on Osteoporosis Prevention, Diagnosis & Therapy (2001). Osteoporosis prevention, diagnosis, and therapy. *JAMA*, 285, 785-95.

Norman AW. (2006). Minireview: vitamin D receptor: new assignments for an already busy receptor. *Endocrinology*, 147, 5542-8.

Nykjaer A, Dragun D, Walther D, Vorum H, Jacobsen C, Herz J, Melsen F, Christensen EI, Willnow TE. (1999). An endocytic pathway essential for renal uptake and activation of the steroid 25-(OH) vitamin D3. *Cell*, 96, 507-15.

Ohyama Y, Hayashi S, Okuda K. (1989). Purification of 25-hydroxyvitamin D3 24-hydroxylase from rat kidney mitochondria. *FEBS Lett.*, 255, 405-8.

Ohyama Y, Noshiro M, Okuda K. (1991). Cloning and expression of cDNA encoding 25-hydroxyvitamin D3 24-hydroxylase. *FEBS Lett.*, 278, 195-8.

Ohyama Y, Yamasaki T. (2004). Eight cytochrome P450s catalyze vitamin D metabolism. *Front Biosci.*, 9, 3007-18.

Ozono K, Liao J, Kerner SA, Scott RA, Pike JW. (1990). The vitamin D-responsive element in the human osteocalcin gene. Association with a nuclear proto-oncogene enhancer. *J Biol Chem.*, 265, 21881-8.

Pálmer HG, Anjos-Afonso F, Carmeliet G, Takeda H, Watt FM. (2008). The vitamin D receptor is a Wnt effector that controls hair follicle differentiation and specifies tumor type in adult epidermis. *PLoS One.*, 3, e1483.

Pálmer HG, González-Sancho JM, Espada J, Berciano MT, Puig I, Baulida J, Quintanilla M, Cano A, de Herreros AG, Lafarga M, Muñoz A. (2001). Vitamin D(3) promotes the differentiation of colon carcinoma cells by the induction of E-cadherin and the inhibition of beta-catenin signaling. *J Cell Biol.*, 154, 369-87.

Papadimitropoulos E, Wells G, Shea B, Gillespie W, Weaver B, Zytaruk N, Cranney A, Adachi J, Tugwell P, Josse R, Greenwood C, Guyatt G; Osteoporosis Methodology Group and The Osteoporosis Research Advisory Group. (2002). Meta-analyses of therapies for postmenopausal osteoporosis. VIII: Meta-analysis of the efficacy of vitamin D treatment in preventing osteoporosis in postmenopausal women. *Endocr Rev.*, 23, 560-9.

Paredes R, Arriagada G, Cruzat F, Villagra A, Olate J, Zaidi K, van Wijnen A, Lian JB, Stein GS, Stein JL, Montecino M. (2004). Bone-specific transcription factor Runx2 interacts with the 1alpha,25-dihydroxyvitamin D3 receptor to up-regulate rat osteocalcin gene expression in osteoblastic cells. *Mol Cell Biol.*, 24, 8847-61.

Rachez C, Suldan Z, Ward J, Chang CP, Burakov D, Erdjument-Bromage H, Tempst P, Freedman LP. (1998). A novel protein complex that interacts with the vitamin D3 receptor in a ligand-dependent manner and enhances VDR transactivation in a cell-free system. *Genes Dev.*, 12, 1787-800.

Rahmaniyan M, Patrick K, Bell NH. (2005). Characterization of recombinant CYP2C11: a vitamin D 25-hydroxylase and 24-hydroxylase. *Am J Physiol Endocrinol Metab.*, 288, E753-60.

Razzaque MS, Sitara D, Taguchi T, St-Arnaud R, Lanske B. (2006). Premature aging-like phenotype in fibroblast growth factor 23 null mice is a vitamin D-mediated process. *FASEB J.*, 20, 720-2.

Rebel A, Basle M, Pouplard A, Malkani K, Filmon R, Lepatezour A. (1981) Towards a viral etiology for Paget's disease of bone. *Metab Bone Dis Relat Res.*, 3, 235-8.

Rochel N, Wurtz JM, Mitschler A, Klaholz B, Moras D. (2000). The crystal structure of the nuclear receptor for vitamin D bound to its natural ligand. *Mol Cell.,* 5, 173-9.

Sakai S, Takaishi H, Matsuzaki K, Kaneko H, Furukawa M, Miyauchi Y, Shiraishi A, Saito K, Tanaka A, Taniguchi T, Suda T, Miyamoto T, Toyama Y. (2009). 1-Alpha, 25-dihydroxy vitamin D(3) inhibits osteoclastogenesis through IFN-beta-dependent NFATc1 suppression. *J Bone Miner Metab.*, May 19.

Shen Q, Christakos S. (2005). The vitamin D receptor, Runx2, and the Notch signaling pathway cooperate in the transcriptional regulation of osteopontin. *J Biol Chem.*, 280, 40589-98.

Shibata T, Shira-Ishi A, Sato T, Masaki T, Masuda A, Hishiya A, Ishikura N, Higashi S, Uchida Y, Saito MO, Ito M, Ogata E, Watanabe K, Ikeda K (2002). Vitamin D hormone inhibits osteoclastogenesis in vivo by decreasing the pool of osteoclast precursors in bone marrow. *J Bone Miner Res.*, 17, 622-9.

Shimada T, Kakitani M, Yamazaki Y, Hasegawa H, Takeuchi Y, Fujita T, Fukumoto S, Tomizuka K, Yamashita T. (2004). Targeted ablation of Fgf23 demonstrates an essential physiological role of FGF23 in phosphate and vitamin D metabolism. *J Clin Invest.*, 113, 561-8.

Shinki T, Shimada H, Wakino S, Anazawa H, Hayashi M, Saruta T, DeLuca HF, Suda T. (1997). *Cloning and expression of rat 25-hydroxyvitamin D3-1alpha-hydroxylase cDNA.* Proc Natl Acad Sci U S A., 94, 12920-5.

Shinkyo R, Sakaki T, Kamakura M, Ohta M, Inouye K. (2004). Metabolism of vitamin D by human microsomal CYP2R1. *Biochem Biophys Res Commun.,* 324, 451-7.

Shiraishi A, Higashi S, Ohkawa H, Kubodera N, Hirasawa T, Ezawa I, Ikeda K, Ogata E. (1999). The advantage of alfacalcidol over vitamin D in the treatment of osteoporosis. *Calcif Tissue Int.*, 65, 311-6.

Shiraishi A, Ito M, Hayakawa N, Kubota N, Kubodera N, Ogata E. (2006). Calcium supplementation does not reproduce the pharmacological efficacy of alfacalcidol for the treatment of osteoporosis in rats. *Calcif Tissue Int.*, 78, 152-61.

Shiraishi A, Takeda S, Masaki T, Higuchi Y, Uchiyama Y, Kubodera N, Sato K, Ikeda K, Nakamura T, Matsumoto T, Ogata E. (2000). Alfacalcidol inhibits bone resorption and stimulates formation in an ovariectomized rat model of osteoporosis: distinct actions from estrogen. *J Bone Miner Res.*, 15, 770-9.

St-Arnaud R, Messerlian S, Moir JM, Omdahl JL, Glorieux FH. (1997). The 25-hydroxyvitamin D 1-alpha-hydroxylase gene maps to the pseudovitamin D-deficiency rickets (PDDR) disease locus. *J Bone Miner Res.*, 12, 1552-9.

Stoye JP, Fenner S, Greenoak GE, Moran C, Coffin JM. (1988). Role of endogenous retroviruses as mutagens: the hairless mutation of mice. *Cell*, 54, 383-91.

Suda T, Takahashi N, Udagawa N, Jimi E, Gillespie MT, Martin TJ. (1999). Modulation of osteoclast differentiation and function by the new members of the tumor necrosis factor receptor and ligand families. *Endocr Rev.*, 20, 345-57.

Tagami T, Lutz WH, Kumar R, Jameson JL. (1998). The interaction of the vitamin D receptor with nuclear receptor corepressors and coactivators. *Biochem Biophys Res Commun.*, 253, 358-63

Takasu H, Sugita A, Uchiyama Y, Katagiri N, Okazaki M, Ogata E, Ikeda K. (2006). c-Fos protein as a target of anti-osteoclastogenic action of vitamin D, and synthesis of new analogs. *J Clin Invest.*, 116, 528-35.

Takayanagi H, Kim S, Koga T, Nishina H, Isshiki M, Yoshida H, Saiura A, Isobe M, Yokochi T, Inoue J, Wagner EF, Mak TW, Kodama T, Taniguchi T. (2002). Induction and activation of the transcription factor NFATc1 (NFAT2) integrate RANKL signaling in terminal differentiation of osteoclasts. *Dev Cell,* 3, 889-901

Takeyama K, Kitanaka S, Sato T, Kobori M, Yanagisawa J, Kato S. (1997) 25-Hydroxyvitamin D3 1alpha-hydroxylase and vitamin D synthesis. *Science*, 277, 1827-30.

Tsujikawa H, Kurotaki Y, Fujimori T, Fukuda K, Nabeshima Y. (2003). Klotho, a gene related to a syndrome resembling human premature aging, functions in a negative regulatory circuit of vitamin D endocrine system. *Mol Endocrinol.*, 17, 2393-403.

Tsukamoto Y, Hanaoka M, Matsuo T, Saruta T, Nomura M, Takahashi Y. (2000). Effect of 22-oxacalcitriol on bone histology of hemodialyzed patients with severe secondary hyperparathyroidism. *Am J Kidney Dis.*, 35, 458-64.

Uchiyama Y, HiguchI Y, Takeda S, Masaki T, Shira-Ishi A, Sato K, Kubodera N, Ikeda K, Ogata E. (2002). ED-71, a vitamin D analog, is a more potent inhibitor of bone resorption than alfacalcidol in an estrogen-deficient rat model of osteoporosis. *Bone.*, 30, 582-8.

Urakawa I, Yamazaki Y, Shimada T, Iijima K, Hasegawa H, Okawa K, Fujita T, Fukumoto S, Yamashita T. (2006). Klotho converts canonical FGF receptor into a specific receptor for FGF23. *Nature*, 444, 770-4.

Yagishita N, Yamamoto Y, Yoshizawa T, Sekine K, Uematsu Y, Murayama H, Nagai Y, Krezel W, Chambon P, Matsumoto T, Kato S. (2001). Aberrant growth plate development in VDR/RXR gamma double null mutant mice. *Endocrinology*, 142, 5332-41.

Yamagata M, Ozono K, Hashimoto Y, Miyauchi Y, Kondou H, Michigami T. (2005). Intraperitoneal administration of recombinant receptor-associated protein causes phosphaturia via an alteration in subcellular distribution of the renal sodium phosphate co-transporter. *J Am Soc Nephrol.*, 16, 2338-45.

Yamamoto K, Masuno H, Choi M, Nakashima K, Taga T, Ooizumi H, Umesono K, Sicinska W, VanHooke J, DeLuca HF, Yamada S. (2000). *Three-dimensional modeling of and ligand docking to vitamin D receptor ligand binding domain.* Proc Natl Acad Sci U S A., 97, 1467-72.

Yanagisawa J, Yanagi Y, Masuhiro Y, Suzawa M, Watanabe M, Kashiwagi K, Toriyabe T, Kawabata M, Miyazono K, Kato S. (1999). Convergence of transforming growth factor-beta and vitamin D signaling pathways on SMAD transcriptional coactivators. *Science*, 283, 1317-21.

Yoshizawa T, Handa Y, Uematsu Y, Takeda S, Sekine K, Yoshihara Y, Kawakami T, Arioka K, Sato H, Uchiyama Y, Masushige S, Fukamizu A, Matsumoto T, Kato S. (1997). Mice lacking the vitamin D receptor exhibit impaired bone formation, uterine hypoplasia and growth retardation after weaning. *Nat Genet.,* 16, 391-6.

Zhang C, Baudino TA, Dowd DR, Tokumaru H, Wang W, MacDonald PN. (2001) . Ternary complexes and cooperative interplay between NCoA-62/Ski-interacting protein and steroid receptor coactivators in vitamin D receptor-mediated transcription. *J Biol Chem.*, 276, 40614-20.

Zierold C, Darwish HM, DeLuca HF. (1994). *Identification of a vitamin D-response element in the rat calcidiol* (25-hydroxyvitamin D3) 24-hydroxylase gene. Proc Natl Acad Sci U S A., 91, 900-2.

In: Vitamin D: Biochemistry, Nutrition ... ISBN: 978-1-61668-273-6
Editor: W. J. Stackhouse, pp. 129-146

Chapter 5

VITAMIN D AND THE THYROID

***Shannon Wakeley*[*] *and Whitney Goldner*[‡]**
University of Nebraska Medical Center, Omaha, NE, USA

ABSTRACT

Vitamin D deficiency has been implicated in the pathogenesis of several disease processes ranging from autoimmune disease to malignancy. Knowledge in the area of vitamin D deficiency has grown exponentially over recent years, and relationships between vitamin D and many disease conditions, including benign and malignant thyroid disease, have been discovered. Thyroid tissue expresses vitamin D receptors and *in vitro* studies have shown that 1,25$(OH)_2$D (calcitriol) decreases proliferation and increases markers of differentiation in thyroid cancer cells. Vitamin D deficiency has also been found to have direct effects on thyroid function, playing a role in autoimmune hypo- and hyperthyroidism. This chapter will review the role of vitamin D in the thyroid by specifically looking at the function of vitamin D at the cellular level and its effects in both benign and malignant thyroid disease.

* Corresponding Author Address:Whitney Goldner, MD, 983020 Nebraska Medical Center, Omaha, NE 68198-3020, Phone: 402-559-3579, Fax: 402-559-9504, Email: wgoldner@unmc.edu
‡ wgoldner@unmc.edu

INTRODUCTION

The importance of vitamin D in bone mineral homeostasis, skeletal integrity, and the regulation of calcium and phosphorus transport are established (1). However, recent information (2,3) has shown that vitamin D affects more than just bone and mineral metabolism. Some of these effects include regulation of cell differentiation, proliferation and apoptosis in several tumor cells (4,5), modulation of autoimmune disease such as multiple sclerosis, rheumatoid arthritis and type 1 diabetes (6), as well as effects on cardiovascular health (7). Little information is known about vitamin D and the thyroid, specifically the role of vitamin D in thyroid cancer, thyroid nodules and autoimmune thyroid disease. This chapter will review vitamin D metabolism and action with special focus on intrathyroidal vitamin D metabolism and action, polymorphisms of vitamin D enzymes and receptors, the role of vitamin D in thyroid disorders and the effects of vitamin D therapy.

VITAMIN D METABOLISM

$1,25(OH)_2D$ (calcitriol) is the hormonally active form of vitamin D. Synthesis of $1,25(OH)_2D$ involves several steps (Figure 1) (8). Vitamin D_3 (cholecalciferol) is ingested via dietary sources or formed by the photoconversion of 7-dehydrocholesterol in the skin. Vitamin D_2 (ergocalciferol) is formed from UV irradiation of ergosterol obtained from yeast (9,10). Both vitamin D_2 and vitamin D_3 are hydroxylated in the liver by the enzyme vitamin D 25-hydroxylase, encoded by the gene CYP27A1, to form 25(OH)D. 25(OH)D is again hydroxylated to form $1,25(OH)_2D$ via the renal enzyme 25(OH)D-1-α-hydroxylase, encoded by the gene CYP27B1 (3). $1,25(OH)_2D$ is the active form of vitamin D and exerts its biological effects by binding to the nuclear vitamin D receptor (VDR) and forming a heterodimer with the retinoid X receptor (9). Measurement of serum 25(OH)D levels are used to determine a patient's vitamin D status, as 25(OH)D reflects the amount of vitamin D stores in the body (11). Historically there has been controversy regarding the optimal level of 25(OH)D, however, it is now generally accepted that individuals with levels less than 20 ng/mL are vitamin D deficient, 21-29 ng/mL are vitamin D insufficient, and greater than 30 ng/mL have sufficient levels (2).

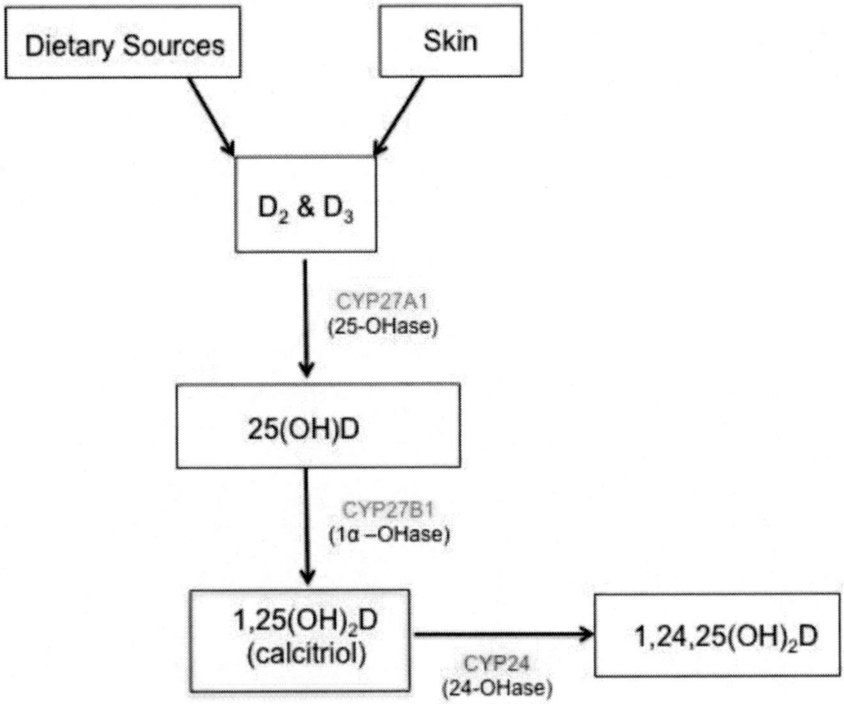

Figure 1. Vitamin D Metabolism

Catabolism of 1,25$(OH)_2$D to its inactive form, 1,24,25$(OH)_2$D, occurs via the enzyme 25-hydroxyvitamin D 24-hydroxylase, encoded by the gene CYP24 (6). Regulation of 1,25$(OH)_2$D concentration is tightly controlled by multiple positive and negative feedback processes (Figure 2) (5). An increase of 1,25$(OH)_2$D, calcium, or phosphate will induce the expression of CYP24 to produce the inactive metabolite 1,24,25$(OH)_2$D, whereas an increase in 1,24,25$(OH)_2$D induces the synthesis of 1,25$(OH)_2$D. CYP27A1 and CYP27B1 expression are induced by parathyroid hormone and suppressed by 1,25$(OH)_2$D (3).

Previously it was thought that CYP27A1 was located only in the liver and CYP27B1 only in the kidney. However, CYP27A1 has since been found in melanoma cells (12), colon cancer cells (13), and fibroblasts (14), and CYP27B1 has been found in at least ten extrarenal cells which include the colon, pancreas, prostate, breast, ovary, placenta, brain, vasculature, macrophages, dendritic cells, parathyroid and thyroid cells (15-19). Vitamin D receptors have been found in thirty-six tissues, including the thyroid (20). This suggests that in the presence of adequate amounts of 25(OH) D, cells in tissues containing CYP27A1, CYP27B1 and vitamin D receptors have the potential to produce biological response.

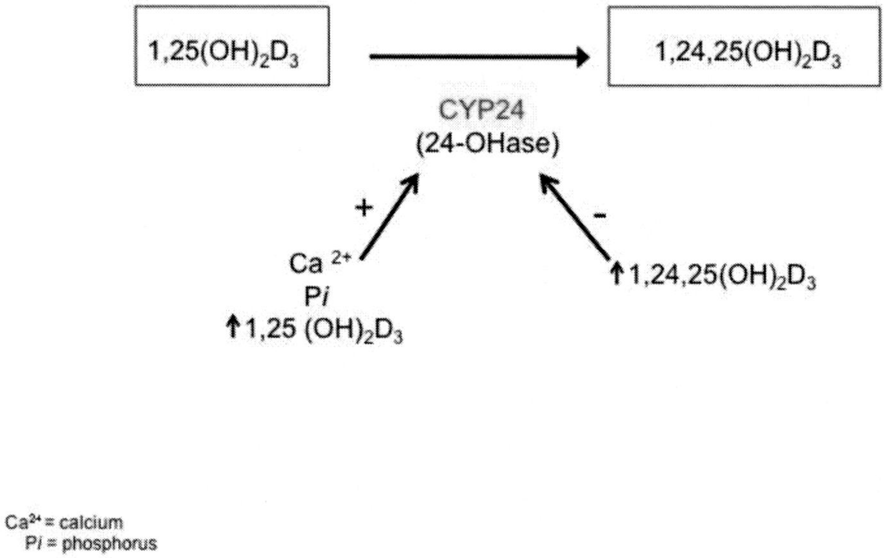

Figure 2. Regulation of $1,25(OH)_2D_3$

Outside the kidney, CYP27B1 appears to be subject to different regulation than the renal enzyme and has a paracrine or autocrine function to augment local production of $1,25(OH)_2D$(3). Therefore, cells containing CYP27B1 are able to produce local concentrations of $1,25(OH)_2D$, generating biological responses at a cellular level (10). Historically, the role of vitamin D had been limited to its physiological regulation of calcium and phosphate transport and bone mineralization (3). However, $1,25(OH)_2D$ has since been shown to have other attributes (21), such as immunomodulation and anti-cancer properties. Not only does vitamin D deficiency have negative implications for bone health, but it could impact other tissues that rely on vitamin D through local production of $1,25(OH)_2D$ via the CYP27B1 enzyme. Research has shown $1,25(OH)_2D$ can down regulate CYP27B1 via negative feedback on vitamin D response elements located on the CYP27B1 gene (22), and that down regulation of CYP27B1 is both tissue and cell type specific. The ability of prostate cancer (23) and colon cancer (24) cells to locally produce $1,25(OH)_2D$ to promote cell differentiation are examples representative of the potential biological importance of vitamin D (10). The specific regulation of vitamin D metabolism in thyroid cells has not yet been elucidated.

VITAMIN D AND CANCER

Vitamin D deficiency has been implicated in the pathogenesis of many cancers, including prostate (25), breast (26), pancreatic (27), colon (28), melanoma (29) and squamous cell carcinomas (30). Several epidemiological studies have revealed an inverse relationship between UVB exposure and incidence of colorectal (31), breast (32) and prostate (33) cancer. An inverse relationship between 25(OH)D levels and the risk of distal colon and rectal cancer was observed in a sub-analysis of patients from the Nurses' Health Study (34). Most normal cells, and many cancerous cells, express vitamin D receptors (16) and vitamin D has several potential therapeutic properties in these cancers (35). It has also been reported that $1,25(OH)_2D$ has actions in cancer cells. These actions include inhibition of proliferation, induction of differentiation, reduction of invasiveness and angiogenesis, and enhanced apoptosis (36-41).

Many cancer cells not only have vitamin D receptors, but they also contain CYP27A1 and CYP27B1, the enzymes necessary to metabolize inactive vitamin D into the hormonally active $1,25(OH)_2D$. CYP27B1 is expressed in extra-renal sites such as normal colon, lymph nodes, brain, pancreas, placenta and skin (16) thereby allowing local production of $1,25(OH)_2D$. Increased CYP27B1 expression has also been observed in breast (42) and prostate (43) cancer but decreased in poorly differentiated colon carcinomas (44,45). Upregulation of CYP24 and downregulation of CYP27B1 has been observed in high-grade colon carcinomas (46). Therefore, defects in the ability of cancer cells to make or maintain hormonally active $1,25(OH)_2D$ have been theorized to play a role in the pathogenesis of poorly differentiated cancers (3).

Because $1,25(OH)_2D$ is inactivated by CYP24 it has been hypothesized that upregulation of CYP24 is the mechanism for increased inactivation of $1,25(OH)_2D$ and subsequent cancer pathogenesis. Expression of CYP24 has been shown to be upregulated in several tumors including breast (47), colon (46), and lung cancers (48). While normal human prostate cells are practically devoid of CYP24, cancer cells have constitutive expression of CYP24 (49). CYP24 is frequently expressed in non-small cell lung cancer but not in the nontumorigenic bronchial epithelial cells. One group demonstrated CYP24 expression using RT-PCR in ten of eighteen primary lung tumors but in only one of eleven normal lung tissue specimens (50), supporting the hypothesis that inactivation of $1,25(OH)_2D$ by CYP24 could modulate or contribute to tumor growth.

VITAMIN D IN THYROID CANCER

Thyroid cancer is the most common endocrine malignancy, being responsible for more deaths than all other endocrine malignancies combined (51). The incidence of thyroid cancer has risen over the past twenty years (51), however there is no consensus as to why this has occurred. Whether it is due to detection bias versus other factors remains unknown. Thyroid cancer cells exhibit wide variations in differentiation. The most differentiated cancers are papillary thyroid carcinoma and follicular thyroid carcinoma, and the least differentiated, and most lethal, is anaplastic thyroid carcinoma (51).

Currently there is no clear clinical association between vitamin D deficiency and thyroid cancer. However, one study showed that individuals with papillary and follicular thyroid cancer had significantly lower levels of circulating $1,25(OH)_2D$ compared to controls (52). Expression of CYP27B1 and vitamin D receptors have been shown in both normal thyroid follicular cells as well as papillary and anaplastic thyroid cancer and CYP24 expression has been demonstrated in anaplastic thyroid cancer cell lines (53,54). When compared to normal thyroid follicular cells, vitamin D receptors and CYP27B1 expression were both increased in papillary thyroid cancer cells as measured by immunohistochemical staining of thyroid tissue (54). Interestingly, the expression of vitamin D receptors varies even amongst tumors of the same subtype (53). When looking at subtypes of thyroid cancer, TPC1 (papillary) and BCPAP (papillary) cells were shown to have increased vitamin D receptor expression as compared to K1 cells (papillary). In addition to variable expression of vitamin D receptors, the presence of certain vitamin D receptor polymorphisms (specifically the haplotype *Tabf*) appeared to be associated with an increased risk of follicular thyroid cancer (52).

In vitro administration of $1,25(OH)_2D$ has been shown to increase expression of the tumor suppressor protein p27 and decrease cell proliferation in cultured papillary and follicular thyroid carcinoma cell lines (55). The increased expression of p27 correlated with decreased metastatic spread. The same group went on to demonstrate that *in vivo* calcitriol administration could restore p27 accumulation in metastatic follicular thyroid carcinoma cells, an effect associated with an appreciably enhanced cellular differentiation, reduction in tumor burden, and prevention of metastatic growth (56). Likewise, the addition of 1,25$(OH)_2$D to UO126, a MAP-kinase inhibitor, showed additive effects toward decreasing viable cell number in TPC1 (papillary), HTH74 (anaplastic), and SW1736 (anaplastic) cell lines (53).

Similar to other cancers, inactivation of 1,25(OH)2D by CYP24 may play a role in cancer pathogenesis by eliminating the beneficial anti-cancer effects of 1,25$(OH)_2$D. Several mechanisms exist to regulate the level of CYP24, one of which is posttranscriptional modification by micro RNA (miRNA). Low levels of miRNA125b result in higher levels of CYP24 (57). Interestingly, significantly lower levels of miRNA125b have been found in anaplastic thyroid cancer compared to normal thyroid tissue (58). It is unknown whether or not CYP24 is differentially expressed in other thyroid cancers, including papillary or follicular thyroid cancer or whether it varies amongst tumor subtypes.

Vitamin D and Thyroid Nodules

Thyroid nodules are common and frequently benign, carrying a 5% risk of malignancy (59). The exact etiology of thyroid nodules is unknown, but prevalence is higher in women, the elderly, and in individuals with history of head or neck radiation exposure or iodine deficiency (60,61). Studies evaluating the direct relationship of vitamin D and thyroid nodules are lacking. However, one study found that rates of vitamin D deficiency were not statistically different between thyroid nodules and active thyroid cancer and thyroid cancer in remission, although the rates were higher in all three groups compared with the general population (62). While previous reports of vitamin D deficiency in healthy populations have ranged from 14-34% (63-65), the rates of vitamin D deficiency in nodules was 48%, thyroid cancer in remission was 56% and active thyroid cancer was 58% (62). Whether or not this finding suggests vitamin D deficiency plays a role in the transformation of benign thyroid nodules into malignant nodules is unknown. Further research is needed to evaluate the potential relationship between both benign and malignant nodules as well as the mechanisms responsible if a relationship is found. One potential reason for the elevated rate of vitamin D deficiency in the nodule population compared with healthy controls could be due to the presence of concurrent autoimmune thyroid disease in patients with thyroid nodules.

VITAMIN D AND AUTOIMMUNE DISEASE

Vitamin D has many immunomodulatory properties playing a role in both innate and adaptive immunity (66). $1{,}25(OH)_2D$ has been shown to suppress production of interleukin (IL)-12, IL-2, tumor necrosis factor-α, and λ-interferon cytokines; to activate expression of transforming growth factor-β1 and IL-4 cytokines, thereby inhibiting Th1-type responses and inducing regulatory T-cells (67) One of the first observations linking vitamin D with the immune system was the finding that macrophages were able to synthesize $1{,}25(OH)_2D$ from 25(OH)D (68). It is now known that several cells possess the ability to synthesize $1{,}25(OH)_2D$ (69) leading to observations that intracellular metabolism of $1{,}25(OH)_2D$ can play a role in immunomodulation. Several autoimmune diseases have been linked to vitamin D deficiency including type 1 diabetes (70), rheumatoid arthritis (71), systemic lupus erythematosis (72), and multiple sclerosis (73).

Type 1 diabetes results from autoimmune destruction of pancreatic β-cells resulting in insulin deficiency. It has been associated with lower serum concentrations of $1{,}25(OH)_2D$ and 25(OH)D (74). A Finnish study of 10,366 children showed that vitamin D supplementation in the first year of life reduced the risk of type 1 diabetes by up to 80% (75). The exact mechanism for the development of type 1 diabetes is unknown and likely multifactorial. Another study found evidence that a polymorphism of CYP27B1, common C allele, was associated with type 1 diabetes (76), suggesting defects in metabolizing $1{,}25(OH)_2D$ in addition to vitamin D deficiency play a role in development of type 1 diabetes.

Multiple sclerosis is an autoimmune disease caused by an unknown agent or agents triggering a T-cell mediated inflammatory attack, resulting in demyelination of central nervous tissue (77). There have been many studies linking multiple sclerosis to vitamin D deficiency after it was noted that the prevalence increased in regions with lower ultraviolet B radiation and higher geographical latitudes (78). A large prospective study among 7 million US military personnel showed that higher levels of circulating 25(OH)D were associated with a lower risk of multiple sclerosis. For every 20 ng/mL increase in 25(OH)D, the risk of multiple sclerosis decreased by 41% (77).

Autoimmune disease of the thyroid, the most common cause for thyroid dysfunction, is quite common (79), resulting in hypothyroidism in patients with Hashimoto's thyroiditis (lymphocytic thyroiditis) and hyperthyroidism in individuals with Graves' disease. Given the association of vitamin D and other autoimmune diseases, researchers have begun to evaluate the role of vitamin D in autoimmune thyroid disease.

VITAMIN D IN HYPOTHYROIDISM

Unfortunately, to date there is relatively little information on the relationship between vitamin D and autoimmune thyroid disease. Lymphocytic thyroiditis (Hashimoto's thyroiditis) is the most common etiology of hypothyroidism, due to autoimmune-mediated destruction of the thyroid gland involving apoptosis of thyroid epithelial cells and lymphocytic infiltration of the thyroid tissue (80). Patients with Hashimoto's disease have antibodies to thyroglobulin (TG Ab) and thyroid peroxidase (TPO Ab). The exact cause of Hashimoto's disease is unknown, but is thought to be a combination of genetic susceptibility and environmental factors. The role of vitamin D in hypothyroidism has been studied at multiple levels including vitamin D deficiency, vitamin D metabolism, and defects at the vitamin D receptor.

After an *in vitro* study showed additive immunosuppressive effects of $1,25(OH)_2D$ and cyclosporine, a murine model was used to investigate their effects on autoimmune thyroiditis. Mice treated simultaneously with both drugs exhibited a lower incidence of thyroid pathology and developed significantly milder disease, as defined histologically by mononuclear cell thyroid infiltration. When administered alone, $1,25(OH)_2D$ exhibited immunosuppressive properties as opposed to no effect when cyclosporine was given alone (81).

In a study looking at vitamin D levels in persons with autoimmune hypothyroidism, the mean 25(OH)D levels among individuals 33 ± 13.5 years of age was 17 nmol/l (6.8 ng/mL). After controlling for age, there was a significant inverse correlation between 25(OH)D levels and thyroid autoimmunity as reflected by TPO Ab titres (82).

Gene polymorphisms of CYP27B1, the enzyme responsible for converting 25(OH)D to $1,25(OH)_2D$ have also been reported. Because many tissues express CYP27B1, a defect in the ability of this enzyme to function would impair synthesis of $1,25(OH)_2D$. This polymorphism was investigated in patients with Graves' disease, Hashimoto's thyroiditis and type 1 diabetes mellitus, however, no association was found (83). Conversely, investigation of vitamin D receptor gene variants in a Croatian population found that common haplotypic variants within the vitamin D receptor gene 3'-region previously linked to vitamin D receptor mRNA expression and allelic imbalance may be associated with Hashimoto's thyroiditis (84).

VITAMIN D IN HYPERTHYROIDISM

The immunomodulatory effects of $1,25(OH)_2D$ are mediated through the vitamin D receptor. Studies have shown an association between vitamin D receptor gene polymorphisms and the susceptibility to Graves' disease (85). In Taiwanese Chinese patients the vitamin D receptor FokI T/C polymorphism was associated with a higher prevalence of Graves' disease (86). In addition to the vitamin D receptor FokI gene region, vitamin D receptor BsmI and ApaI gene regions were associated with Graves' disease in a study of Japanese patients (87). Vitamin D receptor gene polymorphisms have also been found in German and Polish populations, FokI variant "f" and BSMI variant "b" respectively, however none were found in Serbian or UK Caucasian populations (85,88).

A mouse model studying the effect of vitamin D on Graves' hyperthyroidism found that mice deprived of vitamin D in their diet had lower levels of T4 prior to induction of Graves' and had persistent hyperthyroidism after induction of Graves' was achieved by thyrotropin receptor immunization (89). Although this suggests vitamin D deficiency plays a role in Graves' disease, conclusive evidence of this has not been demonstrated in animal models or humans.

CONCLUSION

There is evidence that vitamin D plays a role in the pathogenesis of thyroid disease, however more research is needed to define the exact mechanisms. It is clear that $1,25(OH)_2D$ has several immunomodulatory properties affecting both thyroid autoimmune disease and thyroid cancer. Understanding what factors play a role in the metabolism of $1,25(OH)_2D$ as well as action at the level of the vitamin D receptor will be necessary to potentiate the beneficial actions of $1,25(OH)_2D$.

REFERENCES

[1] Holick MF. Vitamin D and bone health. *J.Nutr.* 1996 Apr;126(4 Suppl):1159S-64S.

[2] Stechschulte SA, Kirsner RS, Federman DG. Vitamin D: bone and beyond, rationale and recommendations for supplementation. *Am.J.Med.* 2009 Sep;122(9):793-802.

[3] Deeb KK, Trump DL, Johnson CS. Vitamin D signalling pathways in cancer: potential for anticancer therapeutics. *Nat.Rev.Cancer.* 2007 Sep;7(9):684-700.

[4] Ordonez-Moran P, Larriba MJ, Pendas-Franco N, Aguilera O, Gonzalez-Sancho JM, Munoz A. Vitamin D and cancer: an update of in vitro and in vivo data. *Front.Biosci.* 2005 Sep 1;10:2723-2749.

[5] Hansen CM, Binderup L, Hamberg KJ, Carlberg C. Vitamin D and cancer: effects of 1,25(OH)2D3 and its analogs on growth control and tumorigenesis. *Front.Biosci.* 2001 Jul 1;6:D820-48.

[6] DeLuca HF. Evolution of our understanding of vitamin D. *Nutr.Rev.* 2008 Oct;66(10 Suppl 2):S73-87.

[7] Gouni-Berthold I, Krone W, Berthold HK. Vitamin D and cardiovascular disease. *Curr.Vasc.Pharmacol.* 2009 Jul;7(3):414-422.

[8] Bringhurst F, Demay M, Kronenberg H. *Hormones and disorders of Mineral Metabolism.* 11th ed. Philadelphia, PA: Saunders Elsevier; 2008. p. 1217.

[9] Prentice A, Goldberg GR, Schoenmakers I. Vitamin D across the lifecycle: physiology and biomarkers. *Am.J.Clin.Nutr.* 2008 Aug;88(2):500S-506S.

[10] Norman AW. From vitamin D to hormone D: fundamentals of the vitamin D endocrine system essential for good health. *Am.J.Clin.Nutr.* 2008 Aug;88(2):491S-499S.

[11] Pilz S, Tomaschitz A, Obermayer-Pietsch B, Dobnig H, Pieber TR. Epidemiology of vitamin D insufficiency and cancer mortality. *Anticancer Res.* 2009 Sep;29(9):3699-3704.

[12] Reichrath J, Rech M, Moeini M, Meese E, Tilgen W, Seifert M. In vitro comparison of the vitamin D endocrine system in 1,25(OH)2D3-responsive and -resistant melanoma cells. *Cancer.Biol.Ther.* 2007 Jan;6(1):48-55.

[13] Matusiak D, Benya RV. CYP27A1 and CYP24 expression as a function of malignant transformation in the colon. *J.Histochem.Cytochem.* 2007 Dec;55(12):1257-1264.

[14] Ellfolk M, Norlin M, Gyllensten K, Wikvall K. Regulation of human vitamin D(3) 25-hydroxylases in dermal fibroblasts and prostate cancer LNCaP cells. *Mol.Pharmacol.* 2009 Jun;75(6):1392-1399.
[15] Stolzenberg-Solomon RZ. Vitamin D and pancreatic cancer. *Ann.Epidemiol.* 2009 Feb;19(2):89-95.
[16] Zehnder D, Bland R, Williams MC, McNinch RW, Howie AJ, Stewart PM, et al. Extrarenal expression of 25-hydroxyvitamin d(3)-1 alpha-hydroxylase. *J.Clin.Endocrinol.Metab.* 2001 Feb;86(2):888-894.
[17] Hewison M, Freeman L, Hughes SV, Evans KN, Bland R, Eliopoulos AG, et al. Differential regulation of vitamin D receptor and its ligand in human monocyte-derived dendritic cells. *J.Immunol.* 2003 Jun 1;170(11):5382-5390.
[18] Zehnder D, Bland R, Chana RS, Wheeler DC, Howie AJ, Williams MC, et al. Synthesis of 1,25-dihydroxyvitamin D(3) by human endothelial cells is regulated by inflammatory cytokines: a novel autocrine determinant of vascular cell adhesion. *J.Am.Soc.Nephrol.* 2002 Mar;13(3):621-629.
[19] Zehnder D, Bland R, Walker EA, Bradwell AR, Howie AJ, Hewison M, et al. Expression of 25-hydroxyvitamin D3-1alpha-hydroxylase in the human kidney. *J.Am.Soc.Nephrol.* 1999 Dec;10(12):2465-2473.
[20] Bouillon R, Okamura WH, Norman AW. Structure-function relationships in the vitamin D endocrine system. *Endocr.Rev.* 1995 Apr;16(2):200-257.
[21] Nagpal S, Na S, Rathnachalam R. Noncalcemic actions of vitamin D receptor ligands. *Endocr.Rev.* 2005 Aug;26(5):662-687.
[22] Turunen MM, Dunlop TW, Carlberg C, Vaisanen S. Selective use of multiple vitamin D response elements underlies the 1 alpha,25-dihydroxyvitamin D3-mediated negative regulation of the human CYP27B1 gene. *Nucleic Acids Res.* 2007;35(8):2734-2747.
[23] Moreno J, Krishnan AV, Feldman D. Molecular mechanisms mediating the anti-proliferative effects of Vitamin D in prostate cancer. *J.Steroid Biochem.Mol.Biol.* 2005 Oct;97(1-2):31-36.
[24] Cross HS, Kallay E, Khorchide M, Lechner D. Regulation of extrarenal synthesis of 1,25-dihydroxyvitamin D3--relevance for colonic cancer prevention and therapy. *Mol.Aspects Med.* 2003 Dec;24(6):459-465.
[25] Ahonen MH, Tenkanen L, Teppo L, Hakama M, Tuohimaa P. Prostate cancer risk and prediagnostic serum 25-hydroxyvitamin D levels (Finland). *Cancer Causes Control* 2000 Oct;11(9):847-852.

[26] Bertone-Johnson ER, Chen WY, Holick MF, Hollis BW, Colditz GA, Willett WC, et al. Plasma 25-hydroxyvitamin D and 1,25-dihydroxyvitamin D and risk of breast cancer. *Cancer Epidemiol.Biomarkers Prev.* 2005 Aug;14(8):1991-1997.
[27] Chiang KC, Chen TC. Vitamin D for the prevention and treatment of pancreatic cancer. *World J.Gastroenterol.* 2009 Jul 21;15(27):3349-3354.
[28] Garland CF, Comstock GW, Garland FC, Helsing KJ, Shaw EK, Gorham ED. Serum 25-hydroxyvitamin D and colon cancer: eight-year prospective study. *Lancet* 1989 Nov 18;2(8673):1176-1178.
[29] Nurnberg B, Graber S, Gartner B, Geisel J, Pfohler C, Schadendorf D, et al. Reduced serum 25-hydroxyvitamin D levels in stage IV melanoma patients. *Anticancer Res.* 2009 Sep;29(9):3669-3674.
[30] Lipworth L, Rossi M, McLaughlin JK, Negri E, Talamini R, Levi F, et al. Dietary vitamin D and cancers of the oral cavity and esophagus. *Ann.Oncol.* 2009 Sep;20(9):1576-1581.
[31] Garland CF, Garland FC. Do sunlight and vitamin D reduce the likelihood of colon cancer? *Int.J.Epidemiol.* 1980 Sep;9(3):227-231.
[32] Gorham ED, Garland FC, Garland CF. Sunlight and breast cancer incidence in the USSR. *Int.J.Epidemiol.* 1990 Dec;19(4):820-824.
[33] Schwartz GG, Hulka BS. Is vitamin D deficiency a risk factor for prostate cancer? (Hypothesis). *Anticancer Res.* 1990 Sep-Oct;10(5A):1307-1311.
[34] Feskanich D, Ma J, Fuchs CS, Kirkner GJ, Hankinson SE, Hollis BW, et al. Plasma vitamin D metabolites and risk of colorectal cancer in women. *Cancer Epidemiol.Biomarkers Prev.* 2004 Sep;13(9):1502-1508.
[35] Holick MF. Vitamin D: its role in cancer prevention and treatment. *Prog.Biophys.Mol.Biol.* 2006 Sep;92(1):49-59.
[36] Ylikomi T, Laaksi I, Lou YR, Martikainen P, Miettinen S, Pennanen P, et al. Antiproliferative action of vitamin D. *Vitam.Horm.* 2002;64:357-406.
[37] Wang X, Studzinski GP. Activation of extracellular signal-regulated kinases (ERKs) defines the first phase of 1,25-dihydroxyvitamin D3-induced differentiation of HL60 cells. *J.Cell.Biochem.* 2001;80(4):471-482.
[38] Mantell DJ, Owens PE, Bundred NJ, Mawer EB, Canfield AE. 1 alpha,25-dihydroxyvitamin D(3) inhibits angiogenesis in vitro and in vivo. *Circ.Res.* 2000 Aug 4;87(3):214-220.

[39] Simboli-Campbell M, Narvaez CJ, van Weelden K, Tenniswood M, Welsh J. Comparative effects of 1,25(OH)2D3 and EB1089 on cell cycle kinetics and apoptosis in MCF-7 breast cancer cells. *Breast Cancer Res.Treat.* 1997 Jan;42(1):31-41.

[40] Liu M, Lee MH, Cohen M, Bommakanti M, Freedman LP. Transcriptional activation of the Cdk inhibitor p21 by vitamin D3 leads to the induced differentiation of the myelomonocytic cell line U937. *Genes Dev.* 1996 Jan 15;10(2):142-153.

[41] Shabahang M, Buras RR, Davoodi F, Schumaker LM, Nauta RJ, Evans SR. 1,25-Dihydroxyvitamin D3 receptor as a marker of human colon carcinoma cell line differentiation and growth inhibition. *Cancer Res.* 1993 Aug 15;53(16):3712-3718.

[42] Townsend K, Banwell CM, Guy M, Colston KW, Mansi JL, Stewart PM, et al. Autocrine metabolism of vitamin D in normal and malignant breast tissue. *Clin.Cancer Res.* 2005 May 1;11(9):3579-3586.

[43] Schwartz GG, Whitlatch LW, Chen TC, Lokeshwar BL, Holick MF. Human prostate cells synthesize 1,25-dihydroxyvitamin D3 from 25-hydroxyvitamin D3. *Cancer Epidemiol.Biomarkers Prev.* 1998 May;7(5):391-395.

[44] Bareis P, Bises G, Bischof MG, Cross HS, Peterlik M. 25-Hydroxy-Vitamin D Metabolism in Human Colon Cancer Cells during Tumor Progression. *Biochem.Biophys.Res.Commun.* 2001 Jul 27;285(4):1012-1017.

[45] Bises G, Kallay E, Weiland T, Wrba F, Wenzl E, Bonner E, et al. 25-hydroxyvitamin D3-1alpha-hydroxylase expression in normal and malignant human colon. *J.Histochem.Cytochem.* 2004 Jul;52(7):985-989.

[46] Cross HS, Bises G, Lechner D, Manhardt T, Kallay E. The Vitamin D endocrine system of the gut--its possible role in colorectal cancer prevention. *J.Steroid Biochem.Mol.Biol.* 2005 Oct;97(1-2):121-128.

[47] Friedrich M, Rafi L, Mitschele T, Tilgen W, Schmidt W, Reichrath J. Analysis of the vitamin D system in cervical carcinomas, breast cancer and ovarian cancer. Recent Results *Cancer Res.* 2003;164:239-246.

[48] Anderson MG, Nakane M, Ruan X, Kroeger PE, Wu-Wong JR. Expression of VDR and CYP24A1 mRNA in human tumors. *Cancer Chemother.Pharmacol.* 2006 Jan;57(2):234-240.

[49] Khorchide M, Lechner D, Cross HS. Epigenetic regulation of vitamin D hydroxylase expression and activity in normal and malignant human prostate cells. *J.Steroid Biochem.Mol.Biol.* 2005 Feb;93(2-5):167-172.

[50] Parise RA, Egorin MJ, Kanterewicz B, Taimi M, Petkovich M, Lew AM, et al. CYP24, the enzyme that catabolizes the antiproliferative agent vitamin D, is increased in lung cancer. *Int.J.Cancer* 2006 Oct 15;119(8):1819-1828.
[51] Cobin RH, Gharib H, Bergman DA, Clark OH, Cooper DS, Daniels GH, et al. AACE/AAES medical/surgical guidelines for clinical practice: management of thyroid carcinoma. American Association of Clinical Endocrinologists. American College of Endocrinology. *Endocr.Pract.* 2001 May-Jun;7(3):202-220.
[52] Penna-Martinez M, Ramos-Lopez E, Stern J, Hinsch N, Hansmann ML, Selkinski I, et al. Vitamin D receptor polymorphisms in differentiated thyroid carcinoma. *Thyroid* 2009 Jun;19(6):623-628.
[53] Sharma V, Fretwell D, Haugen B, Klopper JP. Vitamin D Receptor (VDR) Actiavation Decreases Thyroid Cancer Cell Growth and Is Enhanced by Inhibition of the Mitogen-Activated *Protein Kinase* (MAPK) Pathway. 2009.
[54] Khadzkou K, Buchwald P, Westin G, Dralle H, Akerstrom G, Hellman P. 25-hydroxyvitamin D3 1alpha-hydroxylase and vitamin D receptor expression in papillary thyroid carcinoma. *J.Histochem.Cytochem.* 2006 Mar;54(3):355-361.
[55] Liu W, Asa SL, Fantus IG, Walfish PG, Ezzat S. Vitamin D arrests thyroid carcinoma cell growth and induces p27 dephosphorylation and accumulation through PTEN/akt-dependent and -independent pathways. *Am.J.Pathol.* 2002 Feb;160(2):511-519.
[56] Dackiw AP, Ezzat S, Huang P, Liu W, Asa SL. Vitamin D3 administration induces nuclear p27 accumulation, restores differentiation, and reduces tumor burden in a mouse model of metastatic follicular thyroid cancer. *Endocrinology* 2004 Dec;145(12):5840-5846.
[57] (57) Komagata S, Nakajima M, Takagi S, Mohri T, Taniya T, Yokoi T. Human CYP24 catalyzing the inactivation of calcitriol is post-transcriptionally regulated by miR-125b. *Mol.Pharmacol.* 2009 Jul 1.
[58] (58) Visone R, Pallante P, Vecchione A, Cirombella R, Ferracin M, Ferraro A, et al. Specific microRNAs are downregulated in human thyroid anaplastic carcinomas. *Oncogene* 2007 Nov 29;26(54):7590-7595.
[59] Gharib H, Papini E, Valcavi R, Baskin HJ, Crescenzi A, Dottorini ME, et al. American Association of Clinical Endocrinologists and Associazione Medici Endocrinologi medical guidelines for clinical

practice for the diagnosis and management of thyroid nodules. *Endocr.Pract.* 2006 Jan-Feb;12(1):63-102.

[60] (60) Sherman SI. Thyroid carcinoma. *Lancet* 2003 Feb 8;361(9356):501-511.

[61] Nagataki S, Nystrom E. Epidemiology and primary prevention of thyroid cancer. *Thyroid* 2002 Oct;12(10):889-896.

[62] Laney N, Meza J, Lyden E, Erickson J, Treude K, Goldner W. The Prevalence of Vitamin D Deficiency Is Similar between Thyroid Nodule and Thyroid Cancer Patients. *International Journal of Endocrinology* 2010;vol. 2010,(Article ID 805716, 7 pages, 2010. doi:10.1155/2010/805716):7 pages.

[63] Goldner WS, Stoner JA, Thompson J, Taylor K, Larson L, Erickson J, et al. Prevalence of vitamin D insufficiency and deficiency in morbidly obese patients: a comparison with non-obese controls. *Obes.Surg.* 2008 Feb;18(2):145-150.

[64] Haney EM, Stadler D, Bliziotes MM. Vitamin D insufficiency in internal medicine residents. *Calcif.Tissue Int.* 2005 Jan;76(1):11-16.

[65] Zadshir A, Tareen N, Pan D, Norris K, Martins D. The prevalence of hypovitaminosis D among US adults: data from the NHANES III. *Ethn.Dis.* 2005 Autumn;15(4 Suppl 5):S5-97-101.

[66] Adams JS, Hewison M. Unexpected actions of vitamin D: new perspectives on the regulation of innate and adaptive immunity. *Nat.Clin.Pract.Endocrinol.Metab.* 2008 Feb;4(2):80-90.

[67] Bailey R, Cooper JD, Zeitels L, Smyth DJ, Yang JH, Walker NM, et al. Association of the vitamin D metabolism gene CYP27B1 with type 1 diabetes. *Diabetes* 2007 Oct;56(10):2616-2621.

[68] Adams JS, Sharma OP, Gacad MA, Singer FR. Metabolism of 25-hydroxyvitamin D3 by cultured pulmonary alveolar macrophages in sarcoidosis. *J.Clin.Invest.* 1983 Nov;72(5):1856-1860.

[69] Townsend K, Evans KN, Campbell MJ, Colston KW, Adams JS, Hewison M. Biological actions of extra-renal 25-hydroxyvitamin D-1alpha-hydroxylase and implications for chemoprevention and treatment. *J.Steroid Biochem.Mol.Biol.* 2005 Oct;97(1-2):103-109.

[70] Harris SS. Vitamin D in type 1 diabetes prevention. *J.Nutr.* 2005 Feb;135(2):323-325.

[71] Merlino LA, Curtis J, Mikuls TR, Cerhan JR, Criswell LA, Saag KG, et al. Vitamin D intake is inversely associated with rheumatoid arthritis: results from the Iowa Women's Health Study. *Arthritis Rheum.* 2004 Jan;50(1):72-77.

[72] Kamen D, Aranow C. Vitamin D in systemic lupus erythematosus. *Curr.Opin.Rheumatol.* 2008 Sep;20(5):532-537.

[73] Ponsonby AL, Lucas RM, van der Mei IA. UVR, vitamin D and three autoimmune diseases--multiple sclerosis, type 1 diabetes, rheumatoid arthritis. *Photochem.Photobiol.* 2005 Nov-Dec;81(6):1267-1275.

[74] Pozzilli P, Manfrini S, Crino A, Picardi A, Leomanni C, Cherubini V, et al. Low levels of 25-hydroxyvitamin D3 and 1,25-dihydroxyvitamin D3 in patients with newly diagnosed type 1 diabetes. *Horm.Metab.Res.* 2005 Nov;37(11):680-683.

[75] Hypponen E, Laara E, Reunanen A, Jarvelin MR, Virtanen SM. Intake of vitamin D and risk of type 1 diabetes: a birth-cohort study. *Lancet* 2001 Nov 3;358(9292):1500-1503.

[76] Bailey R, Cooper JD, Zeitels L, Smyth DJ, Yang JH, Walker NM, et al. Association of the vitamin D metabolism gene CYP27B1 with type 1 diabetes. *Diabetes* 2007 Oct;56(10):2616-2621.

[77] Munger KL, Levin LI, Hollis BW, Howard NS, Ascherio A. Serum 25-hydroxyvitamin D levels and risk of multiple sclerosis. *JAMA* 2006 Dec 20;296(23):2832-2838.

[78] Fernandes de Abreu DA, Eyles D, Feron F. Vitamin D, a neuro-immunomodulator: Implications for neurodegenerative and autoimmune diseases. *Psychoneuroendocrinology* 2009 Jun 20.

[79] McGrogan A, Seaman HE, Wright JW, de Vries CS. The incidence of autoimmune thyroid disease: a systematic review of the literature. *Clin.Endocrinol.*(Oxf) 2008 Nov;69(5):687-696.

[80] Cooper DS, Greenspan FS, Ladenson PW. Greenspan's Basic & *Clinical Endocrinology: The Thyroid Gland.* . 8th ed.: McGraw-Hill; 2007.

[81] Fournier C, Gepner P, Sadouk M, Charreire J. In vivo beneficial effects of cyclosporin A and 1,25-dihydroxyvitamin D3 on the induction of experimental autoimmune thyroiditis. *Clin.Immunol.Immunopathol.* 1990 Jan;54(1):53-63.

[82] Goswami R, Marwaha RK, Gupta N, Tandon N, Sreenivas V, Tomar N, et al. Prevalence of vitamin D deficiency and its relationship with thyroid autoimmunity in Asian Indians: a community-based survey. *Br.J.Nutr.* 2009 Aug;102(3):382-386.

[83] Pani MA, Regulla K, Segni M, Krause M, Hofmann S, Hufner M, et al. Vitamin D 1alpha-hydroxylase (CYP1alpha) polymorphism in Graves' disease, Hashimoto's thyroiditis and type 1 diabetes mellitus. *Eur.J.Endocrinol.* 2002 Jun;146(6):777-781.

[84] Stefanic M, Papic S, Suver M, Glavas-Obrovac L, Karner I. Association of vitamin D receptor gene 3'-variants with Hashimoto's thyroiditis in the Croatian population. *Int.J.Immunogenet.* 2008 Apr;35(2):125-131.

[85] Ramos-Lopez E, Kurylowicz A, Bednarczuk T, Paunkovic J, Seidl C, Badenhoop K. Vitamin D receptor polymorphisms are associated with Graves' disease in German and Polish but not in Serbian patients. *Thyroid* 2005 Oct;15(10):1125-1130.

[86] Chen RH, Chang CT, Chen HY, Chen WC, Tsai CH, Tsai FJ. Association between vitamin-D receptor gene FokI polymorphism and Graves' disease among Taiwanese Chinese. J.*Clin.Lab.Ana*l. 2007;21(3):173-177.

[87] Ban Y, Taniyama M, Ban Y. Vitamin D receptor gene polymorphism is associated with Graves' disease in the Japanese population. *J.Clin.Endocrinol.Metab*. 2000 Dec;85(12):4639-4643.

[88] Collins JE, Heward JM, Nithiyananthan R, Nejentsev S, Todd JA, Franklyn JA, et al. Lack of association of the vitamin D receptor gene with Graves' disease in UK Caucasians. *Clin.Endocrinol.*(Oxf) 2004 May;60(5):618-624.

[89] Misharin A, Hewison M, Chen CR, Lagishetty V, Aliesky HA, Mizutori Y, et al. Vitamin D deficiency modulates Graves' hyperthyroidism induced in BALB/c mice by thyrotropin receptor immunization. *Endocrinology* 2009 Feb;150(2):1051-1060.

In: Vitamin D: Biochemistry, Nutrition ... ISBN: 978-1-61668-273-6
Editor: W. J. Stackhouse, pp. 147-166

Chapter 6

EFFECT OF MAGNESIUM DEFICIENCY ON VITAMIN D METABOLISM AND ACTION

***Robert K. Rude*[*a] *and Helen E. Gruber*[b]**
[a]USC Keck School of Medicine and Orthopaedic Hospital, Los Angeles, CA
[b]Department of Orthopaedic Surgery, Carolinas Medical Center, Charlotte, NC

ABSTRACT

Magnesium (Mg) deficiency affects mineral metabolism in a dramatic fashion. Patients with severe Mg deficiency may present with increased neuromuscular hyperexcitablity characterized by paresthesias, muscle cramps and spasm, tetany, and seizures. This is thought to be secondary to profound hypocalcemia and Mg-deficiency induced decreased parathyroid hormone (PTH) secretion and PTH end-organ resistance, although low serum Mg concentrations can produce similar effects without concomitant hypocalcemia. More moderate degrees of Mg deficiency have also been linked to osteoporosis. Serum concentrations of 25(OH)-vitamin D have been observed to be low in patients with severe Mg deficiency and to be resistant to the administration of vitamin D metabolites. Similarly, serum concentrations of $1,25(OH)_2$-vitamin D are

* Corresponding Author: Robert K. Rude, M.D., Orthopaedic Hospital, Endocrinology Research Laboratory, 2400 South Flower Street, Los Angeles, CA 90007, Telephone:213-742-1376, Fax:213-742-1365, Email:rrude60075@aol.com

low in Mg deficiency. Experimental Mg depletion in humans and in animal models has resulted in a fall in serum 1,25$(OH)_2$-vitamin D levels. This paper will review the evidence that Mg deficiency in both humans and in animals does adversely affect vitamin D metabolism and/or action

INTRODUCTION

Calcium and the metabolites of vitamin D, 25-hydroxyvitamin D and 1,25-dihydroxyvitmin D, along with parathyroid hormone play an important role in skeletal metabolism as well as other biological processes. Magnesium is also known to modulate the synthesis and action of these hormones and therefore plays an important role in these same processes. Studies have demonstrated that the usual dietary intake or nutritional status of these factors are suboptimal. This chapter will summarize the prevalence of these deficiencies and review the evidence for the role of magnesium deficiency in the action and/or metabolism of vitamin D and its metabolites.

PREVALENCE OF VITAMIN D DEFICIENCY AND INSUFFICIENCY

Vitamin D deficiency is defined as a serum concentration of 25-hydroxyvitamin D of less than 20 ng/ml, and vitamin D insufficiency is defined by a concentration of less that 30 ng/ml. It is estimated that 40-100% of U.S. and European elderly men and women are vitamin D deficient (1). A recent study of older men in the U.S. demonstrated 26% were vitamin D deficiency and 72% were insufficient in vitamin D (2,3). The incidence of vitamin D insufficiency appears to be increasing rapidly (4). This problem also exists in children (1). A recent study in a population aged 1-21 found 9% were vitamin D deficient and 61% were vitamin D insufficient (5). These data therefore suggest that low vitamin D status may negatively affect skeletal metabolism as well as many other medical problems (1).

PREVALENCE OF CALCIUM DEFICIENCY

Low dietary calcium (Ca) intake is a recognized risk factor for osteoporosis (6-8). Low dietary Ca has been reported to predict bone density as well as fracture rate in some studies (8-10). Dietary Ca intake falls far below the established Adequate Intake (AI) set by the U.S. Food Nutrition Board from adolescence to old age (11). For example, in females the mean Ca intake at age 14-18 is 753 mg/day (AI = 1300 mg), at age 31-50. 590 mg/day (AI = 1000 mg) and at age 51-70, 510 mg/day (AI = 1200 mg). Ca supplements have been shown to enhance bone mass accumulation in adolescence and retard bone loss in later life (12-15). Since peak bone mass is an important predictor of osteoporosis in later life, low Ca intake is particularly critical during adolescence when much of the skeleton is formed (14,15). Ten to twenty percent of adolescent girls have a Ca intake less than 500 mg/day (16). A recent study reported that pubertal girls only partially adapt to low dietary Ca intake thereby placing them at great risk for inadequate Ca retention (16). This inability to adapt may be linked to other nutritional deficiencies, as studies that assess multiple nutrient effects on bone suggest that other dietary factors also impact bone mass (17-19). It is likely that there are substantial detrimental effects on bone when multiple bone-related nutritional deficiencies, such as vitamin D deficiency, are present.

PREVALENCE OF MAGNESIUM DEFICIENCY

Magnesium (Mg), the second most prevalent intracellular cation in the body, plays an important role in enzyme activity, membrane stability and ion transport (20). Mg exists in macronutrient quantities in bone (0.5-1% bone ash) and dietary Mg deficiency has been implicated as a risk factor for osteoporosis (20-23). The U.S. Food Nutrition Board established the RDA for Mg for adult males at 420 mg/day and for adult females at 320 mg/day (24). The usual dietary Mg intake, however, falls below this recommendation.

According to the USDA (25), the mean Mg intake for males is 323 mg/day (81% of the RDA) and the mean intake for females is 228 mg/day (68% of RDA). This deficiency, as with Ca deficiency, is present from adolescence to old age. In females, the mean Mg intake at age 14-18 is 225 mg/day (RDA = 360 mg), at age 31-50, 236 mg/day (RDA = 320 mg), and at age 51-70 , 239 mg/day (RDA = 320mg). This substantial dietary Mg deficit is particularly important in an aging population where gastrointestinal and renal mechanisms for Mg conservation may not be as efficient as in a younger population (26,27). Ten percent of elderly women in the U.S. consume $\leq$ 136 mg of Mg per day. Morbid conditions associated with body Mg loss (diabetes, alcoholism, malabsorption) and medications (diuretics, cyclosporine, aminiglycosides, cisplatin, amphotericin B) also exacerbate this problem (20).

Effect of Magnesium Deficiency on Parathyroid Hormone Secretion and Action

It is known that Mg deficiency, when severe, will markedly disturb Ca homeostasis, resulting in impaired parathyroid hormone (PTH) secretion and PTH end-organ resistance which lead to hypocalcemia and neuromuscular hyperexcitability (20) Acute changes in the serum Mg concentration in normal subjects modulate PTH secretion (similar to Ca) via the Ca^{2+}-sensing receptor. While acute changes in extracellular Mg concentrations will influence PTH secretion in a manner qualitatively similar to calcium, it is clear that Mg deficiency markedly perturbs mineral homeostasis (28-30).

Hypocalcemia is a prominent manifestation of Mg deficiency in humans (28-30) as well as in most other species (30-32). In humans, Mg deficiency must become moderate to severe before symptomatic hypocalcemia develops. Mg therapy alone restores serum Ca concentrations to normal (28). Calcium and/or vitamin D therapy will not correct the hypocalcemia (28, 29).

A major factor resulting in the fall in serum Ca is impaired parathyroid gland function. Determination of serum PTH concentrations in hypocalcemic hypomagnesemic patients has shown that the majority of patients have low or normal serum PTH levels (28,34-36) (Figure 1). Normal serum PTH concentrations are thought to be inappropriately low in the presence of hypocalcemia. Therefore, a state of hypoparathyroidism exists in most hypocalcemic Mg-deficient patients. With Mg therapy, the serum PTH rises to elevated levels within minutes (28). The serum PTH concentration will gradually fall to normal within several days of therapy with return of the serum calcium concentration to normal (28,33,36).

Some Mg deficient patients, however, have elevated levels of serum PTH (28,36,37) The presence of normal or elevated serum concentrations of PTH in the face of hypocalcemia (28,29,36) suggests that there may also be end organ resistance to PTH action. In one study, PTH administration did not result in elevation in the serum Ca concentration or urinary hydroxyproline excretion in hypocalcemic hypomagnesemic patients (38). Following Mg repletion, however, a clear response to PTH was observed. PTH has also been shown to have a reduced calcemic effect in Mg-deficient animals (39-41). In one study of the isolated perfused canine femur, the ability of PTH to simulate an increase in the venous cyclic AMP was impaired during perfusion with low Mg fluid, suggesting skeletal PTH resistance (42).

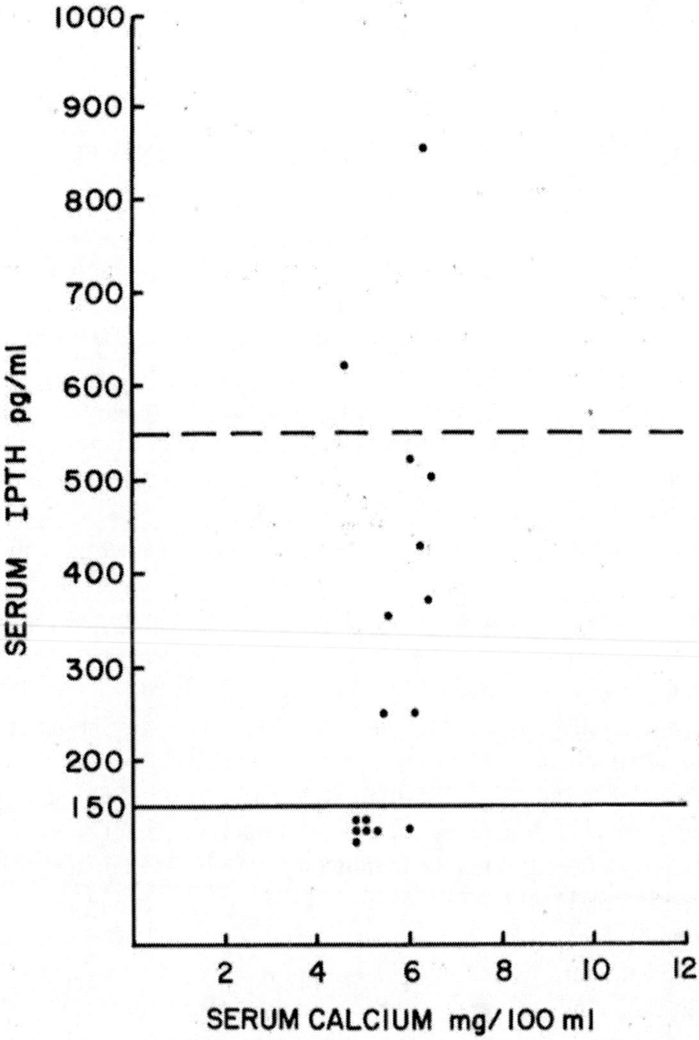

Figure 1. Correlation between the serum PTH concentration with the serum Ca concentration in sixteen hypocalcemic hypomagnesemic patients. The dashed line denotes the upper limit of normal, and the solid line represents the lower level of detection of serum PTH concentration. (Reprinted from reference 28 with permission).

The renal response to PTH has also been assessed by determining the urinary excretion of cyclic AMP and/or phosphate in response to exogenous PTH. Studies in severely Mg-depleted patients demonstrated an impaired response to PTH (28, 29, 38, 43,44). A decrease in urinary cyclic AMP excretion in response to PTH has also been described in the Mg-deficient dog and rat (40,41).

EFFECT OF MAGNESIUM DEFICIENCY ON VITAMIN D METABOLISM AND ACTION

Mg may also be important in vitamin D metabolism and/or action. Patients with hypoparathyroidism, malabsorption syndromes, and rickets have been reported to be resistant to therapeutic doses of vitamin D until Mg was administered simultaneously (29). Patients with hypocalcemia and Mg deficiency have also been reported to be resistant to pharmacological doses of vitamin D (45,46), 1α hydroxyvitamin D (47,48) and 1,25-dihydroxyvitamin D (49). Similarly, an impaired calcemic response to vitamin D has been found in Mg-deficient rats (50), lambs (51), and calves (52).

The exact nature of altered vitamin D metabolism and/or action in Mg deficiency is unclear. Intestinal calcium transport in animal models of Mg deficiency has been found to be reduced in some (53), but not all (54), studies. Calcium malabsorption was associated with low serum levels of 25-hydroxyvitamin D in one study (50), but not in another (54), suggesting that Mg deficiency may impair intestinal Ca absorption by more than one mechanism. Patients with Mg deficiency and hypocalcemia frequently have low serum concentrations of 25-hydroxyvitamin D (55,56), and therefore nutritional vitamin D deficiency may be an important factor in such patients (Figure 2). Therapy with vitamin D, however, results in high serum levels of 25-hydroxyvitamin D without correction of the hypocalcemia (57), suggesting that the vitamin D nutrition is not the major reason. In addition, conversion of radiolabeled vitamin D to 25-hydroxyvitamin D was found to be normal in three Mg-deficient patients (58). Serum concentrations of 1,25-dihydroxyvitamin D have also been found to be low or low normal in most hypocalcemic Mg-deficient patients (30,55,56, 59) (Figure 2). Mg-deficient diabetic children, when given a low Ca diet, did not exhibit the expected normal rise in serum 1,25-dihydroxyvitamin D or PTH (60); the response returned to normal, however, following Mg therapy (61).

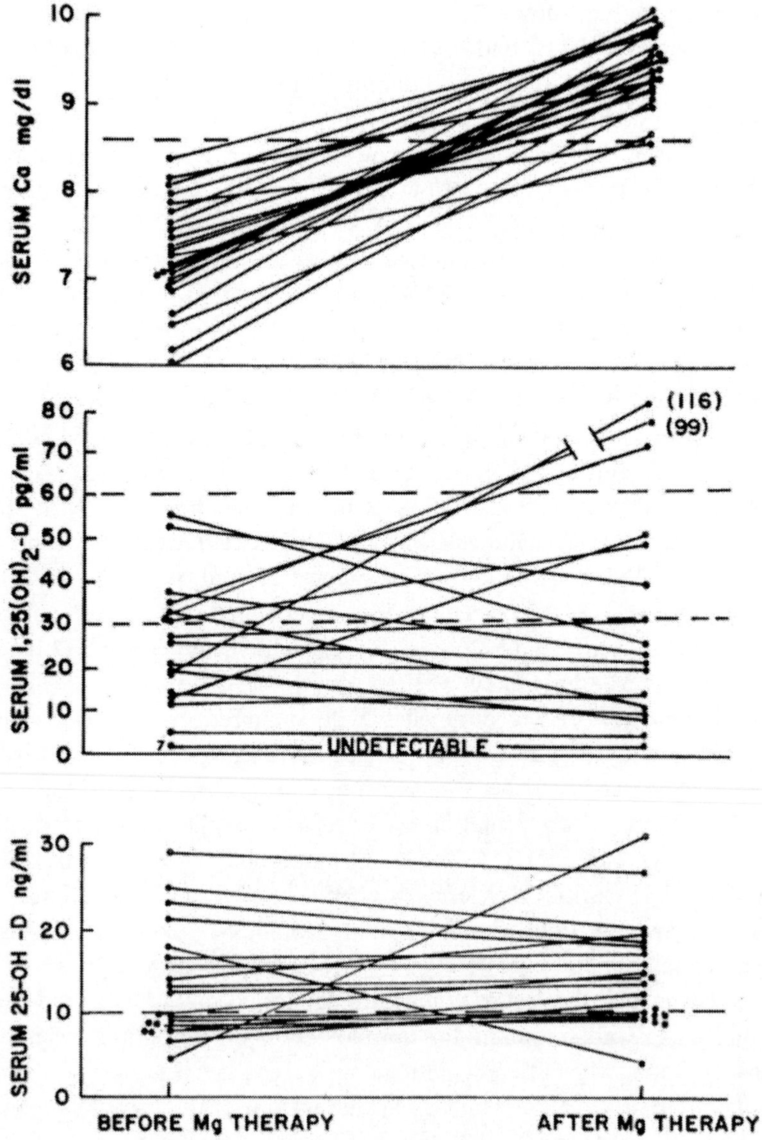

Figure 2. Serum concentrations of Ca, 1,25-dihydroxyvitamin-D and 25-hydroxyvitamin-D in 22 hypocalcemic magnesium-deficient patients before and after 5-8 days of parenteral Mg therapy. The dashed line in the top panel represents the lower normal limit for serum Ca, in the middle panel, the upper and lower limit of normal for serum 1,25-dihydroxyvitamin-D, and in the lower panel, the lower normal limit for 25-hydroxyvitamin D concentrations. (Reprinted from reference 55 with permission).

Recent work has shown that vitamin D insufficient adult women with a blunted response to PTH, had low serum Mg levels (62). Because PTH is a major trophic for 1,25-dihydroxyvitamin D formation, the low serum PTH concentrations could explain the low 1,25-dihydroxyvitamin D levels. In support of this is the finding that some hypocalcemic Mg-deficient patients treated with Mg have a rise in serum 1,25-dihydroxyvitamin D to high normal or to frankly elevated levels, as shown in Figure 2 (55). Most patients, however, do not have a significant rise within one week after institution of Mg therapy, despite a rise in serum PTH and normalization of the serum calcium concentration (Fig. 2) (55). These data suggest that Mg deficiency in humans also impairs the ability of the kidney to synthesize 1,25-dihydroxyvitamin D.

This is supported by the observation that exogenous administration of 1–34 human PTH to normal subjects after 3 weeks of experimental Mg depletion resulted in a significantly lower rise in serum 1,25-dihydroxyvitamin D concentrations than before institution of the diet (see below) (63). It appears, therefore, that the renal synthesis of 1,25-dihydroxyvitamin D is sensitive to Mg depletion. While Mg is known to support 25-hydroxy-1α-hydroxylase *in vitro* (64), the exact Mg requirement for this enzymatic process is not known. Reduced bone-specific binding sites for 1,25-dihydroxyvitamin D have also been reported in Mg deficiency (65).

The association of Mg deficiency with impaired vitamin D metabolism and action therefore may be due to several factors, including vitamin D deficiency (55, 56,65,66) and a decrease in PTH secretion (28,33-36), as well as a direct effect of Mg depletion on the ability of the kidney to synthesize 1,25-dihydroxyvitamin D (55,56,63). Osteoporotic patients with a blunted response to PTH exhibit Mg deficiency (68). In addition, Mg deficiency may directly impair intestinal Ca absorption (28,53,55). Skeletal resistance to vitamin D and its metabolites may also play an important role (47,48-50). It is clear, however, that the restoration of normal serum 1,25-dihydroxyvitamin D concentrations is not required for normalization of the serum calcium level (Figure 2). Most Mg-deficient patients who receive Mg therapy exhibit an immediate rise in PTH, followed by normalization of the serum calcium prior to any change in serum 1,25-dihydroxyvitamin D concentrations (55,56).

EFFECT OF EXPERIMENTAL MAGNESIUM DEPLETION ON SERUM CONCENTRATIONS OF 1,25(OH)$_2$-VITAMIN D IN HUMANS AND ANIMALS

As noted above, Mg deficient patients may have multiple nutritional deficiencies including Ca and vitamin D deficiencies. We therefore conducted experimental human Mg depletion studies by placing 26 normal subjects on a low magnesium diet (12 mg per day) for 21 days. Serum Mg, Ca, PTH and 1,25-dihydroxyvitamin D were determined before and at the conclusion of the dietary period (63). Magnesium depletion was documented by a fall in serum Mg as well as an increase in the retention of an intravenous infusion of magnesium (Figure 3). There was a significant fall in the serum calcium and 1,25-dihydroxyvitamin D as well (Figure 3). The changes observed in PTH were heterogeneous with 20 of the 26 individuals who exhibited no change (n=8) or a fall in serum PTH (n=12) despite the significant decrease in the serum Ca.

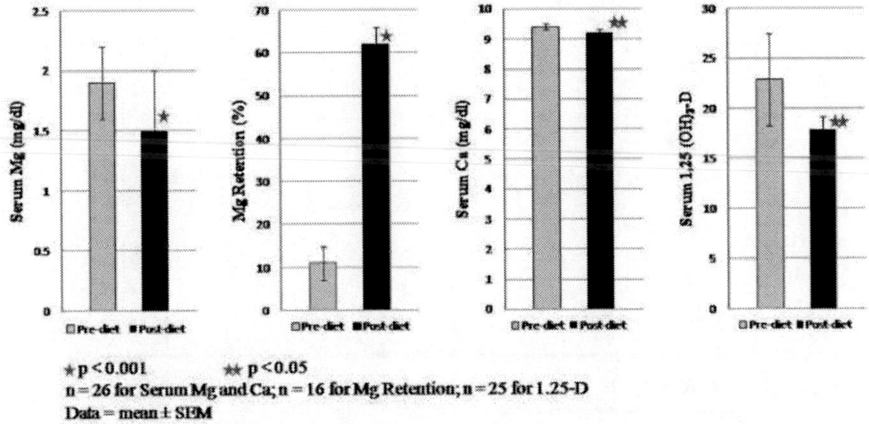

Figure 3. Changes in the serum Mg (n = 26), % Mg retention (n = 16), serum Ca (n = 26, and 1,25-dihydroxyvitamin-D (n = 25) in normal human subjects on a low Mg diet for 21 days. (Adapted from reference 63 with permission).

Renal resistance to PTH was assessed in 13 of the study subjects by determining the serum 1,25-dihydroxyvitamin D concentration before and after a 6 hour PTH infusion pre- and post-diet. As noted in Figure 4, there was a significant fall in serum 1,25-dihydroxyvitamin D in the basal level from pre- to post diet. The rise in serum 1,25-dihydroxyvitamin D in response to the

PTH infusion post diet was significantly lower than pre-diet suggesting a degree of renal resistance had occurred in response to the low magnesium diet.

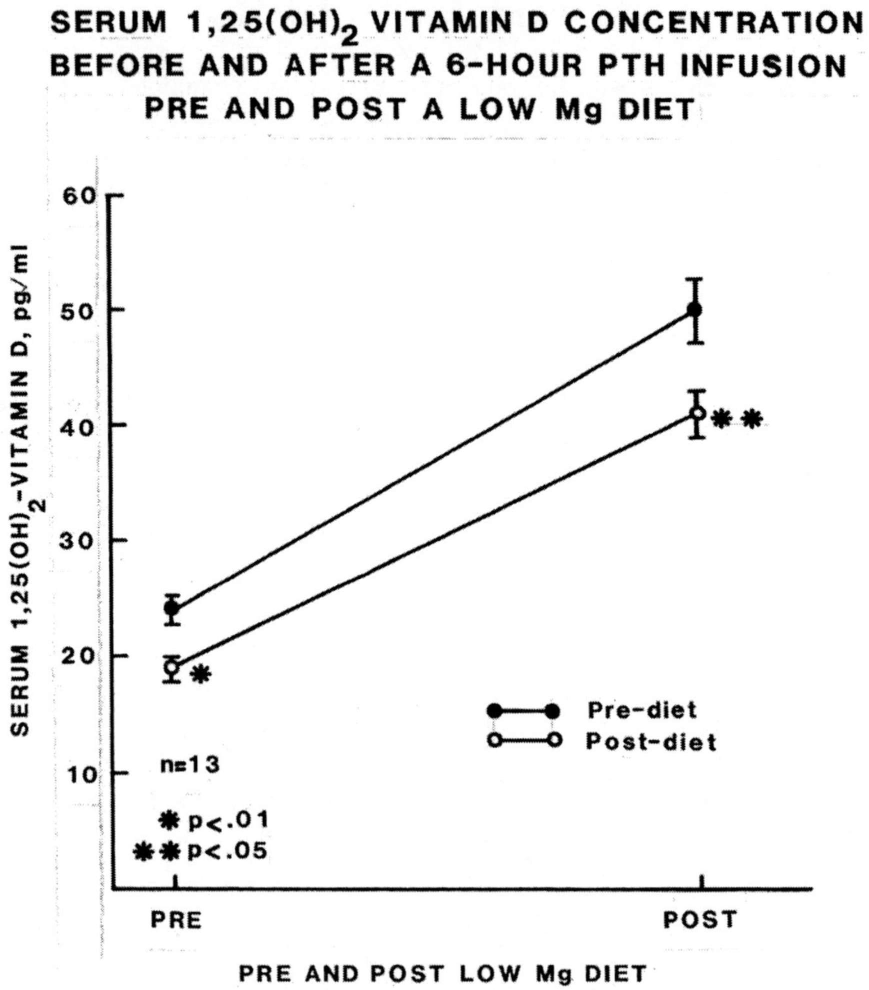

Figure 4. Changes in the serum 1,25-dihydroxyvitamin-D in 13 normal human subjects before and after a low Mg diet for 21 days following a PTH infusion. Data mean ± sem. (Adapted from reference 63 with permission).

The effect of dietary Mg depletion on bone and mineral homeostasis in animals has also been studied, primarily using the rat model. Dietary restriction has usually been severe (0.002 to 0.08 g/Kg diet; normal 0.5 g/Kg diet). A universal observation has been a decrease in growth of both the whole body as well as the skeleton (66-71). Bone from Mg deficient rats has been described as brittle and fragile (72,73). Biomechanical testing has directly demonstrated skeletal fragility in both rat and pig (73-75). Reduction in bone mass compared to control animals occurs in dietary Mg depletion within 6 weeks (71,73-76). We have also observed a decrease in bone mass and a fall in serum 1,25-dihydroxyvitamin D and PTH in rats on a very low Mg diet (0.002% Mg as percent of total diet) as compared to control (0.063% Mg as percent of total diet) as shown in Figures 5 and 6 (76).

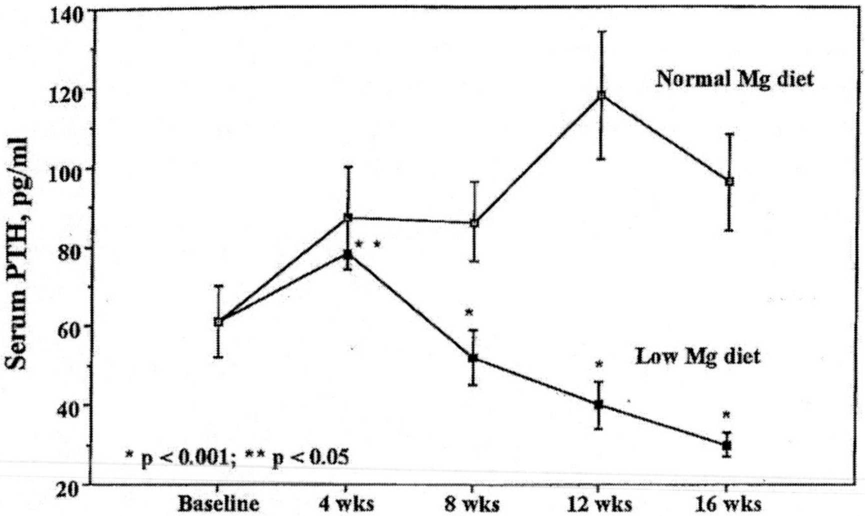

Figure 5. Significant fall in the serum PTH concentration in rats on a very low Mg diet (n = 28) compared to a control diet (n = 34). (Reprinted from reference 76 with permission).

These very low dietary Mg intakes probably do not often occur in the human population. We have, for the first time, studied the effect of less severe dietary Mg restriction on bone metabolism. We employed dietary Mg deprivation in the rat at 10%, 25% and 50% of recommended nutrient (RN) requirement (normal control was 0.05% Mg as percent of total diet) on skeletal metabolism and again found that trabecular bone loss occurred at all these dietary Mg intake levels (77-79). These dietary intake levels reflect similar levels of dietary Mg inadequacy in segments of our population as discussed above. Data for serum determinations at 6 months in the dietary Mg deprivation group are demonstrated in Table 1. It is noted that the serum Mg was significantly lower in the 10% and 25% NR groups but not in the 50% NR group. The serum Ca tended to be slightly higher in the lower Mg diet groups but slightly lower in the 50% group. This is explained by the fact that Ca and Mg appear to share a common intestinal transport system (80), and, in the absence of intestinal dietary Mg, fractional Ca absorption is increased. A low Ca diet will prevent hypercalcemia in the Mg-deficient rodent (81). Therefore, at the 50% Mg diet, the changes in serum Ca are similar to humans and other vertebrates. The serum PTH was lower in the 10% and 25% dietary groups, but at the more mild depletion of 50% of NR was elevated. This could be explained by the fact that Mg is acting in a manner similar to Ca by binding to the calcium-sensing receptor at this higher diet Mg intake. Despite these changes, there was a significant fall in serum 1,25-dihydroxyvitamin D in all groups which demonstrates that Mg deficiency reduces this metabolite of vitamin D regardless of the observed changes in serum Mg, Ca, or PTH. These data again suggest that even moderate degrees of Mg depletion adversely affect vitamin D metabolism.

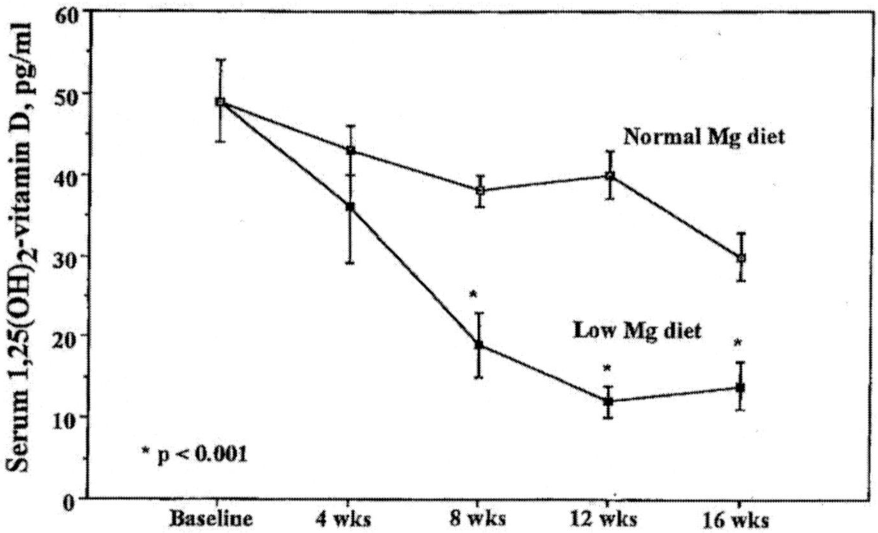

Figure 6. Significant fall in the serum 1,25-dihyroxyvitamin D concentration in rats on a very low Mg diet (n = 28) compared to a control diet (n = 34). (Reprinted from reference 76 with permission).

Table 1. Serum Concentrations of Mg, Ca, PTH, and 1,25(OH)$_2$-Vitamin D in Rats on Low Mg Diets at 10%, 25%, and 50% of Nutritional Requirement (RN) for 6 months.

	10% NR		**25% NR**		**50% NR**	
	Control	**Low Mg**	**Control**	**Low Mg**	**Control**	**Low Mg**
sMg, mg/dl	1.9 ± 0.2	0.6 ± 0.1*	1.6 ± 0.2	0.9 ± 0.2*	2.0 ± 0.2	1.9 ± 0.3
sCa, mg/dl	8.6 ± 0.5	9.9 ± 0.4*	8.5 ± 0.6	9.2 ± 0.6***	10.1 ± 0.6	9.6 ± 0.3$^{\delta}$
sPTH, pg/ml	361 ± 228	141 ± 56**	320 ± 146	134 ± 116$^{\alpha}$	381 ± 281	505 ± 302
s1,25D,pg/ml	18.9 ± 16.6	2.9 ± 0.5**	18.0 ± 13	8.0 ± 4.0$^{\beta}$	23.5 ± 12.7	10.6 ± 7.1**

Data = mean ± SD. * $p<.001$; ** $p<.01$; *** $p< .02$; α $p< .002$; β $p< .05$; δ $p<.004$
n = 12 for Control and Low Mg in 10%, 25%, and 50% dietary groups.
(adapted from data from ref 77, 78, and 79 with permission)

Conclusion

This review demonstrates that Mg deficiency has a profound effect on vitamin D and PTH metabolism and/or action. This interaction probably plays an important role in skeletal health and the increased risk of osteoporosis observed in Mg deficient humans and animals. Assessment of dietary Mg intake, Mg status, and vitamin D and Ca nutrition should be made in patients with osteoporosis.

References

[1] Holick, MF. Vitamin D Deficiency. 2007, *N Engl J Med* 357:266-281.

[2] Orwell, E, Neilson CM, Marshall, LM, Lambert, L, Holton, KF, Hoffman, AR, Barrett-Conner, E, Shikany, JM, Dam, T, and Cauley, JA. Vitamin D deficiency in older men. 2009, *J Clin Endocrinol Metab* 94, 1214-1222.

[3] Holick, MF. MrOs is D-ficient. 2009, *J Clin Endocrinol Metab* 94, 1092-1093.

[4] Ginde, AA, Liu, MC, and Camargo, CA. Demographic differences and trends of vitamin D insufficiency in the US population, 1988-2004. 2009, *Arch Intern Med* 169, 626-632.

[5] Kumar, J, Munter P, Kaskei, FJ, Hailpern, SM, and, Melamed, ML. *Prevalence and associations of 25-hydroxyvitamin D deficiency in US*

children: NHANES 2001-2004. 2009, Pediatrics online (doi:10.1542/peds.2009-0051).

[6] Consensus Development Conference: Prophylaxis and treatment of osteoporosis. 1991, *Am J Med* 90, 107-110.

[7] *Optimal calcium intake.* 1994, NIH Consensus Statement 12:1-24.

[8] Heaney, RP. Calcium, dairy products and osteoporosis. 2000, *J Am Coll Nutr* 19, 83s-99s.

[9] Dawson-Hughes, B, Gallai, GE, Drall, EA, Sadowski, L, Sahyoun N, Tannenbaum, S. A controlled trial of the effect of calcium supplementation on bone density in postmenopausal women. 1990, *N Engl J Med* 323, 878-883.

[10] Meyer HE. Calcium and osteoporotic fractures. 2004, *Br J Nutr* 91, 505-506.

[11] *Dietary Reference Intakes for calcium, phosphorus, magnesium, vitamin D, and fluoride.* 1997, National Academy Press, Washington, D.C., 71-145.

[12] Flynn A. *The role of dietary calcium in bone health.* 2003, Proc Nutr Soc 62, 851-858.

[13] Cashman KD, Flynn A. Optimal nutrition: calcium, magnesium and phosphorus. 1999, *Proc Nutr Soc* 58, 477-487.

[14] Bachrach LK. Acquisition of optimal bone mass in childhood and adolescence. 2001, *Trends Endocrinol Metab* 12, 22-28.

[15] Weaver CM. Calcium and magnesium requirements of children and adolescents and peak bone mass. 2000, *Nutrition* 16, 514-516.

[16] Abrams SA, Griffin IJ, Hicks PD, Gunn SK. Pubertal girls only partially adapt to low dietary calcium intakes. 2004, *J Bone Miner* Res 19, 759-763.

[17] Tranquilli AL, Lucino E, Garzetti GG, Romanini C. Calcium, phosphorus and magnesium intakes correlate with bone mineral content in postmenopausal women. 1994, *Gynecol Endocrinol* 8, 55-58.

[18] New SA, Bolton-Smith C, Grubb DA, Reid DM. Nutritional influences on bone mineral density: A cross-sectional study in premenopausal women. 1997, *Am J Clin Nutr* 65:1831-1839.

[19] Macdonald HM, New SA, Golden MHN, Campbell MK, Reid DM. Nutritional associations with bone loss during the menopausal transition: evidence of a beneficial effect of calcium, alcohol, and fruit and vegetable nutrients and of a detrimental effect of fatty acids. 2004, *Am Soc Clin Nutr* 79, 155-165.

[20] Rude RK. Magnesium Deficiency: a heterogeneous cause of disease in humans. 1998, *J Bone Miner Res* 13, 749-758.
[21] Sojka JE, Weaver CM. Magnesium supplementation and osteoporosis. 1995, *Nutr Rev* 53, 71-80.
[22] Cohen L, Kitzes R. 1981, Infrared spectroscopy and magnesium content of bone mineral in osteoporotic women. *Israel J Med Sci* 17, 1123-1125.
[23] Wallach S. Effects of magnesium on skeletal metabolism. 1990, *Magnes Trace Elem* 9, 1-14.
[24] *Dietary Reference Intakes for calcium, phosphorus, magnesium, vitamin D, and fluoride.* 1997, National Academy Press, Washington, D.C., 190-249.
[25] Cleveland LE, Goldman JD, Borrude LG 1994 Data tables: Results from USDA 1994 continuing survey of food intakes by individuals and 1994 diet and health knowledge survey. *Agricultural Research Service,* U.S. Department of Agriculture, Beltsville, MD.
[26] Lowik MRH, van Dokkum W, Kistemaker C, Schaafasma G, Ockhuizen T. Body composition, health status and urinary magnesium excretion among elderly people (Dutch nutrition surveillance system). 1993, *Magnes Res* 63, 223-232.
[27] Martin BJ. The magnesium load test: Experience in elderly subjects. 1990, *Aging* 2, 291-296.
[28] Rude, R. K., Oldham, S. B., and Singer, F. R. Functional hypoparathyroidism and parathyroid hormone end-organ resistance in human magnesium deficiency. 1976, *Clin. Endocrinol.* 5, 209–224.
[29] Rude, R. K. (1994). Magnesium deficiency in parathyroid function. *In "The Parathyroids"* (J. P. Bilezikian, ed.), pp. 829–842. Raven Press, New York.
[30] Rude, R. K., and Shils, M. E. (2006). *Magnesium. In "Modern Nutrition in Health and Disease"* (M. E. Shils, ed.), pp. 223-247. Lippincott Williams and Wilkins, Philadelphia.
[31] Shils, M. E., Magnesium, calcium and parathyroid hormone interactions. 1980, *Ann. N.Y. Acad. Sci.* 355, 165–180.
[32] Anast, C. S., and Forte, L. F. Parathyroid function and magnesium depletion in the rat. 1983, *Endocrinology* 113, 184–189.
[33] Anast, C. S., Mohs, J. M., Kaplan, S. L., and Burns, T. W. Evidence for parathyroid failure in magnesium deficiency. 1972, *Science* 177, 606–608.

[34] Chase, L. R., and Slatopolsky, E. Secretion and metabolic efficacy of parathyroid hormone in patients with severe hypomagnesemia. 1974, J. *Clin. Endocrinol. Metab.* 38, 363–371.

[35] Suh, S. M., Tashjian, A. H., Matsuo, N., Parkinson, D. K., and Fraser, D. Pathogenesis of hypocalcemia in primary hypomagnesemia: Normal end-organ responsiveness to parathyroid hormone, impaired parathyroid gland function. 1973, *J. Clin. Invest.* 52, 153–160.

[36] Rude, R. K., Oldham, S. B., Sharp, C. F., Jr., and Singer, F. R. Parathyroid hormone secretion in magnesium deficiency. 1978, *J. Clin. Endocrinol. Metab.* 47, 800–806.

[37] Allgrove, J., Adami, S., Fraher, L., Reuben, A., and O'Riordan, J. L. H. Hypomagnesaemia: Studies of parathyroid hormone secretion and function. 1984, *Clin. Endocrinol.* 21, 435–449.

[38] Estep, H., Shaw, W. A., Watlington, C., Hobe, R., Holland, W., and Tucker, S. G. Hypocalcemia due to hypomagnesemia and reversible parathyroid hormone unresponsiveness. 1969, *J. Clin. Endocrinol.* 29, 842–848.

[39] MacManus, J., Heaton, F. W., and Lucas, P. W. A decreased response to parathyroid hormone in magnesium deficiency. 1971, *J. Endocrinol.* 49, 253–258.

[40] Levi, J., Massry, S. G., Coburn, J. W., Llach, F., and Kleeman, C. R. Hypocalcemia in magnesium-depleted dogs: Evidence for reduced responsiveness to parathyroid hormone and relative failure of parathyroid gland function. 1974, *Metabolism* 23, 323–335.

[41] Forbes, R. M., and Parker, H. M. Effect of magnesium deficiency on rat bone and kidney sensitivity to parathyroid hormone.1980, *J. Nutr.* 110, 1610–1617.

[42] Freitag, J. J., Martin, K. J., Conrades, M. B., Bellorin-Font, E., Teitelbaum, S., Klahr, S., and Slatopolsky, E. Evidence for skeletal resistance to parathyroid hormone in magnesium deficiency. 1979, *J. Clin. Invest.* 64, 1238–1244.

[43] Medalle, R., and Waterhouse, C. A magnesium-deficient patient presenting with hypocalcemia and hyperphosphatemia. 1973, *Ann. Int. Med.* 79, 76–79.

[44] Mihara, M., Kamikubo, K., Hiramatsu, K., Itaya, S., Ogawa, T., and Sakata, S. Renal refractoriness to phosphaturic action of parathyroid hormone in a patient with hypomagnesemia. 1995, *Intern. Med.* 34, 666-669.

[45] Medalle, R., Waterhouse, C., and Hahn, T. J. Vitamin D resistance in magnesium deficiency. 1976, *Am. J. Clin. Nutr.* 29, 854–858.
[46] Leicht, E., Biro, G., Keck, E., and Langer, H. J. Die hypomagnesiaemie-bedingte hypocalciaemie: funktioneller hypoparathyreoidismus, parathormon-und vitamin D resistenz. 1990, *Klin. Wochenschr.* 68, 678–684.
[47] Ralston, S., Boyle, I. T., Cowan, R. A., Crean, G. P., Jenkins, A., and Thomson, W. S. PTH and vitamin D responses during treatment of hypomagnesaemic hypoparathyroidism. 1983, *Acta Endocrinol.* 103, 535–538.
[48] Selby, P. L., Peacock, M., and Bambach, C. P. Hypomagnesaemia after small bowel resection: Treatment with 1 α-hydroxylated vitamin D metabolites. 1984, *Br. J. Surg.* 71, 334–337.
[49] Graber, M. L., and Schulman, G. Hypomagnesemic hypocalcemia independent of parathyroid hormone. 1986, *Ann. Int. Med.* 104, 804–806.
[50] Lifshitz, F., Harrison, H. C., and Harrison, H. E. Response to vitamin D of magnesium deficient rats.1967, *Proc. Soc. Exp. Biol. Med.* 125, 472–476.
[51] McAleese, D. M., and Forbes, R. M. Experimental production of magnesium deficiency in lambs on a diet containing roughage. 1959, *Nature* 184, 2025–2026.
[52] Smith, R. H. Calcium and magnesium metabolism in calves. 2. Effect of dietary vitamin D and ultraviolet irradiation on milk-fed calves. 1958, *Biochem. J.* 70, 201-205.
[53] Higuchi, J., and Lukert, B. Effects of magnesium depletion on vitamin D metabolism and intestinal calcium transport. 1974, *Clin. Res.* 22, 617.
[54] Coburn, J. W., Reddy, C. R., Brickman, A. S., Hartenbower, D. L., and Friedler, R. M. Vitamin D metabolism in magnesium deficiency. 1975, *Clin. Res.* 23, 3933.
[55] Rude, R. K., Adams, J. S., Ryzen, E., Endres, D. B., Niimi, H., Horst, R. L., Haddad, J. F., and Singer, F. R. Low serum concentrations of 1,25-dihydroxyvitamin D in human magnesium deficiency. 1985, *J. Clin. Endocrinol. Metab.* 61, 933–940.
[56] Fuss, M., Bergmann, P., Bergans, A., Bagon, J., Cogan, E., Pepersack, T., Van Gossum, M., and Corvilain, J. Correction of low circulating levels of 1,25-dihydroxyvitamin D by 25-hydroxyvitamin D during reversal of hypomagnesaemia. 1989, *Clin. Endocrinol.* 31, 31–38.

[57] Medalle, R., Waterhouse, C., and Hahn, T. J. Vitamin D resistance in magnesium deficiency. 1976, *Am. J. Clin. Nutr.* 29, 854–858.

[58] Lukert, B. P. (1980). Effect of magnesium depletion on vitamin D metabolism in man. *In "Magnesium in Health and Disease"* (M. Cantin and M. S. Seelig, eds.), pp. 275–279 Spectrum, New York.

[59] Leicht, E., Schmidt-Gayk, N., Langer, H. J., Sniege, N., and Biro, G. Hypomagnesaemia-induced hypocalcaemia: Concentrations of parathyroid hormone, prolactin and 1,25-dihydroxyvitamin D during magnesium replenishment. 1992, *Magnes. Res.* 5, 33–36.

[60] Saggese, G., Bertelloni, S., Baroncelli, G. I., Federico, G., Calisti, I., and Fusaro, C. (1988). Bone demineralization and impaired mineral metabolism in insulin-dependent diabetes mellitus. *Helv. Paediat. Acta* 43, 405–414.

[61] Saggese, G., Federico, G., Bertelloni, S., Baroncelli, G. I., and Calisti, L. (1991). Hypomagnesemia and the parathyroid hormone-vitamin D endocrine system in children with insulin-dependent diabetes mellitus: Effects of magnesium administration. *J. Pediatr.* 118, 220–225.

[62] Gunnarsson, O, Indridason, OS, Lranzon, L, and Sigurdsson, G. Factors associated with elevater or blunted PTH response in vitamin D insufficient adults. 2008, *J Intern Med.*265, 488-495.

[63] Fatemi, S., Ryzen, E., Flores, J., Endres, D. B., and Rude, R. K. Effect of experimental human magnesium depletion on parathyroid hormone secretion and 1,25-dihydroxyvitamin D metabolism. 1991, *J. Clin. Endocrinol. Metab.* 73, 1067–1072.

[64] Fisco, F., and Traba, M. L. Influence of magnesium on the in vitro synthesis of 24,25-dihydroxyvitamin D3 and 1α,25-dihydroxyvitamin D3. 1992*, Magnes. Res.* 5, 5–14.

[65] Risco, F. and Traba, M.I. Bone specific binding sites for 1,25(OH)-D_3 in magnesium deficiency. 2004, *J. Physiol. Biochem.* 60, 199-204.

[66] Carpenter, T. O. Disturbances of vitamin D metabolism and action during clinical and experimental magnesium deficiency. 1988, *Magnes. Res.* 1, 131–139.

[67] Leicht, E., and Biro, G. Mechanisms of hypocalcaemia in the clinical form of severe magnesium deficit in the human. 1992, *Magnes. Res.* 5, 37–44.

[68] Sahota, O., Mundey M. K., San, P., Godher, I. M., and Hosking, D. J. Vitamin D insufficiency and the blunted PTH response in established osteoporosis: the role of magnesium deficiency. 2006, *Osteoporos. Int.* 17, 1013-1021.

[69] Kenney, MA, McCoy, H, and Williams, L. Effects of magnesium deficiency on strength, mass and composition of rat femur. 1994, *Calcif Tissue Int* 54:44-49.

[70] Mirra, JM, Alcock, NW, Shils, ME, and Tannenbaum, P. Effects of calcium and magnesium deficiencies on rat skeletal development and parathyroid gland area. 1982, *Magnesium* 1:16-33.

[71] Carpenter, TO, Mackowiak, SJ, Troiano, N, aand Gundberg, CM. Osteocalcin and its message: Relationship to bone histology in magnesium-deprived rats. 1992, *Am J Physiol* 263:E107-E114.

[72] Lai, CC, Singer L, and Armstrong ,WD. Bone composition and phosphatase activity in magnesium deficiency in rats. 1975*J Bone Joint Surg* 57, 516-522.

[73] Kenney, MA, McCoy, H, and Williams, L. Effects of dietary magnesium and nickel on growth and bone characteristics in rats. 1992, *J Am Col Nutr* 11:687-693.

[74] Miller ER, Ullrey DE, Zutaut CL, Baltzer BV, Schmidt DA, Hoefer JA, Luecke RW. Magnesium requirement of the baby pig. *J Nutr* 85:13-20, 1965.

[75] Heroux, O, Peter, D, and Tanner, A. Effect of a chronic suboptimal intake of magnesium on magnesium and calcium content of bone and on bone strength of the rat. 1974, *Can J Physiol Pharmacol* 53:304-310.

[76] Rude, RK, Kirchen ,ME, Gruber, HE, Meyer ,MH, Luck, JS, and Crawford, DL. Magnesium deficiency-induced osteoporosis in the rat: Uncoupling of bone formation and bone resorption. 1999, *Magnes Res* 12:257-267.

[77] Rude, RK, Gruber, HE, Norton, HJ, Wei, LY, Frausto, A, and Mills, BG. Bone loss induced by dietary magnesium reduction to 10% Nutrient Requirement in rats is associated with increase release of substance P and tumor necrosis factor-a. 2004, *J Nutr* 134:79-85.

[78] Rude, RK, Gruber, HE, Norton, HJ, Wei, LY, Frausto, A, and Kilburn ' J. Dietary Magnesium Reduction to 25% of Nutrient Requirement Disrupts Bone and Mineral Metabolism in the Rat. 2005, *Bone* 37: 211-219.

[79] Rude, RK, Gruber, HE, Norton ,HJ, Wei, LY, Frausto, A, and Kilburn, J. Reduction of dietary magnesium by only 50% in the rat disrupts bone and mineral metabolism. 2006, *Osteopor Int 1*7: 1022-1032.

[80] Rude RK: *Magnesium Homeostasis*. In: Principles of Bone Biology (3nd edition; Bilezikian JB, Raisz L, Rodan G [editors]). Academic Press, San Diego, CA, pp487–358-513, 2008.

[81] Rude RK, Gruber HE, Wei LY, Frausto A, Mills BG. 2003. Magnesium deficiency: effect on bone and mineral metabolism in the mouse. *Calcif Tiss Int* 72:32–41.

In: Vitamin D: Biochemistry, Nutrition ... ISBN: 978-1-61668-273-6
Editor: W. J. Stackhouse, pp. 167-181

Chapter 7

IMMUNE MECHANISMS BY WHICH TOPICALLY APPLIED VITAMIN D ACTS AS A THERAPEUTIC AGENT

Shelley Gorman* and Prue H. Hart.
University of Western Australia, Perth, Western Australia, Australia

ABSTRACT

Topical creams containing vitamin D derivatives or analogues (calcitriol, calcipotriene) are currently used to treat different skin conditions including psoriasis and vitiligo with some success. The skin diseases that can be treated by topical vitamin D are characterised by irregular proliferation and differentiation of keratinocytes accompanied by inflammation and an influx of immune effector cells. We are now starting to better understand the mechanisms by which vitamin D applied to the skin affects keratinocyte growth and reduces the inflammation and immune responses, which drive these and other diseases. Here we outline some of the processes by which vitamin D modulates inflammatory processes that occur in diseased skin, and immune mechanisms that may be activated by vitamin D in the skin and draining lymphatic tissue to control inappropriate inflammatory responses. In particular, we focus on

* Corresponding Author: Dr Shelley Gorman, Telethon Institute for Child Health Research, Centre for Child Health Research, University of Western Australia, PO Box 855, West Perth, Western Australia, 6872, Australia, email: shelleyg@ichr.uwa.edu.au, phone: +61 8 9489 7884, fax: +61 8 9489 7700

the cell-driven immune responses mediated by keratinocytes, dendritic cells and T cells that may be targets of vitamin D.

INTRODUCTION

Vitamin D is an essential hormone synthesised in the skin following the exposure of skin to the UVB wavelengths present in sunlight. The active form of vitamin D, calcitriol (1,25-dihydroxyvitamin D_3, $1,25(OH)_2D_3$), and analogues of this hormone (eg. calcipotriol, calcipotriene) are successful treatment options for patients with skin diseases such as psoriasis [reviewed by 1]. In a recent clinical trial, calicitriol ointment (3 μg/g) significantly improved psoriasis symptoms in 136 patients treated over 52 weeks where symptoms were assessed by an investigator-rated global severity score [2]. Currently, vitamin D is administered topically as a cream directly to diseased skin. The mode by which vitamin D reduces the morbidity of psoriasis and other inflammatory skin diseases may occur in part by inhibiting the proliferation and inducing the differentiation of keratinocytes in psoriatic lesions [reviewed by 1]. Alternatively, topically applied vitamin D can have effects on immune responses, which may govern the pathogenesis of psoriasis and other inflammatory diseases of the skin. In this review we concentrate on describing the effects that topical vitamin D has on immune cells and responses in the skin and skin-draining lymph nodes.

DISEASES MODIFIED AND POTENTIAL SIDE EFFECTS OF TOPICAL VITAMIN D

Topical vitamin D has been used to treat many skin diseases other than psoriasis that are associated with abnormal keratinocyte proliferation and differentiation [reviewed by 1,3]. In contrast, topical calcipotriol has no affect on the severity of some skin diseases including alopecia totalis, alopecia areata, acne vulgaris and others [reviewed by 3]. Therapy with topical vitamin D has few reported detrimental effects in patients, with no described systemic adverse effects [reviewed by 1]. Studies with radioactively labelled calcitriol (3 μg/g, twice-weekly for 4 weeks) indicate that very little calcitriol applied to the skin is absorbed into the bloodstream [4]. In other investigations, calcitriol (3 μg/g) administered to the skin of patients for 52 [2] or 78 weeks [5] had no significant effects on various parameters used to test for calcium homeostasis. Some of the known side effects of topical vitamin D treatment of psoriasis include skin irritation, itch and erythema [6]. In particular, topical administration of the vitamin D analogue calcipotriol has been associated with an increased number of adverse skin reactions compared to other topical treatments including calcitriol or corticosteroids [6].

EFFECTS OF TOPICAL VITAMIN D ON KERATINOCYTES AND SKIN CELLS

Keratinocyte Proliferation and Differentiation are Modified by Topical Vitamin D

Skin treatment with vitamin D may control psoriasis pathogenesis by inhibiting proliferation and stimulating the differentiation of keratinocytes [reviewed by 1]. The vitamin D receptor (VDR) is expressed by keratinocytes and other cells of the skin (including epithelial cells, Langerhans cells and dermal fibroblasts), and the expression of the VDR regulates the genomic effects of $1,25(OH)_2D_3$ and its analogues [3]. The expression of the VDR was significantly increased in epidermal basal keratinocytes of lesional psoriatic skin following topical calcipotriol treatment [7]. Topical calcitriol reduces the proliferation of keratinocytes and epidermal cells in psoriatic plaques [8,9]. Interestingly, low concentrations of $1,25(OH)_2D_3$ can accelerate keratinocyte growth, while doses $>10^{-8}$ M suppress the proliferation of these cells [10]. Keratinocyte differentiation is also modified by topical calcipotriol or calcitriol as demonstrated by altered expression of keratin proteins [8,11] and other markers of differentiation [9]. In keratinocytes, a number of different genes can be influenced by $1,25(OH)_2D_3$ including those enzymes which regulate $1,25(OH)_2D_3$ synthesis (eg. Cyp24A1). $1,25(OH)_2D_3$ has regulatory activity on networks of genes which have been implicated in the growth, differentiation, inflammation and wound-healing in keratinocytes [reviewed by 3].

Topical Vitamin D 'Normalizes' Psoriatic Skin

The integrity of psoriatic skin can be affected by topical calcipotriol. The expression of adhesion and integrin molecules was 'normalised' to levels in non-psoriatic skin of five patients treated for 8-24 weeks with topical calcipotriol [12]. Other effects of topical 1,25$(OH)_2D_3$, include epidermal thickening and wrinkling of hairless (HR/ICR) mice treated daily for six weeks with 1,25$(OH)_2D_3$ [13]. Transepidermal water loss may be transiently affected by calcipotriol, 1,25$(OH)_2D_3$ or 1,24$(OH)_2D_3$ treatment of hairless mouse skin [14]. However, transepidermal water loss was not modified by topical calcipotriol treatment of human volunteers in which skin irritation was induced by sodium dodecyl sulphate [15].

Topical Vitamin D Regulates Inflammation and Antimicrobial Activity in Psoriatic Skin

The anti-inflammatory effects of topical vitamin D have been highlighted in a recent study, where calcipotriol treatment of psoriatic skin reduced the expression of proinflammatory alarmins (and antimicrobial peptides) β-defensin (HBD) 2 and HBD3 [16]. In the same study, calcipotriol 'normalised' proinflammatory cytokine levels and reduced IL-17A, IL-17F and IL-8 transcript expression in lesional psoriatic skin. In contrast, expression of the antimicrobial cathelicidin was increased by calcipotriol [16]. The active antimicrobial activity of cathelicidin is found in the LL-37 peptide component of the protein. LL-37 is over-expressed in lesional psoriatic skin [16,17]. LL-37 through TLR9 activation increases the ability of plasmacytoid dendritic cells (DC) to secrete type I interferons in response to self-DNA [17]. The ability of topical vitamin D to increase cathelicidin expression may have pro-inflammatory effects on plasmacytotoid DC present in psoriatic skin. However, 1,25$(OH)_2D_3$ does not directly modulate type I interferon production by plasmacytoid DC isolated from peripheral blood of human volunteers [18]. Thus, the role that vitamin D-induced cathelicidin has in modulating psoriatic skin disease is uncertain. In summary, with reduced proinflammatory alarmin and cytokine levels in psoriatic skin, the overall effects of topical vitamin D are anti-inflammatory.

Immune Modifying Mechanisms of Topical Vitamin D

An alternate pathway whereby topical vitamin D reduces skin inflammation is by regulating cells of the immune system, which reside both in the skin, and skin-draining lymph nodes (SDLN). Topical $1,25(OH)_2D_3$ may modify the migration of immune cells into inflamed skin. In addition, topical $1,25(OH)_2D_3$ affects DC and T cells, which are immune cells that modulate adaptive immune responses. Topical $1,25(OH)_2D_3$ may also alter mucosal antibody responses.

Topical Vitamin D Regulates Immune Cell Infiltration into Psoriatic Lesions

Topical calcitriol can alter the accumulation of immune cells within psoriatic plaques. Twice-daily treatment with calcitriol for 4 weeks reduced the proportion of T cells and neutrophils in both the dermis and epidermis of 10 patients with psoriasis [7]. These observations conflict with a report that human T cells treated with $1,25(OH)_2D_3$ (10 nM) *in vitro* upregulate the chemokine receptor CCR10 and have an enhanced capacity to migrate towards the skin-trophic chemokine CCL27 [19]. $1,25(OH)_2D_3$ (~40 nM) treatment *in vitro* also reduced the ability of murine CD4+ T cells to migrate towards stromal cell-derived factor-1 (CXCL12) [20]. Topical application of mice with $1,25(OH)_2D_3$ or calicpotriol (1667 ng/day for 4 days) increased thymic stromal lymphopoietin (TSLP) transcripts in skin and TSLP protein in serum [21]. Continued skin treatment for up to 16 days with $1,25(OH)_2D_3$ or calicpotriol induced an atopic dermatitis-like syndrome characterized by an influx of inflammatory cells into the ears including eosinophils, CD4+ T cells, CD11c+ DC and mast cells and increased secretion of both Th1 and Th2 cytokines [21]. From these studies, it is clear that topically-applied $1,25(OH)_2D_3$ has effects on the migration of cells into the skin site to which $1,25(OH)_2D_3$ is applied; however, these unresolved results suggest that factors such as dose and timing of vitamin D application may affect inflammatory cell migration into diseased skin.

Regulation of Skin-Derived Dendritic Cells by Topical Vitamin D

Topical $1,25(OH)_2D_3$ regulates skin-derived DC such as Langerhans cells. Skin DC density and phenotype was assessed in the ear skin of BALB/c mice, which were administered $1,25(OH)_2D_3$ (400 ng/day) once a day for seven days [22]. The dendritic morphology of MHC classII+ cells (putative skin DC) was reduced by 1,25(OH)$_2$D$_3$ with cells becoming rounded 24 h after the final skin treatment. Treatment of ear skin with 1,25(OH)$_2$D$_3$ significantly reduced the number of MHC classII+ cells at that site by 50% [22]. These observations have recently been repeated following the chronic treatment of mouse skin with topical calcipotriol [23]. Application of calcipotriol cream to normal human skin for four days resulted in a dose-dependent decrease in the number of CD1a+ cells with a dendritic morphology and in the number of dendrites per cell [24].

The reduction in skin DC numbers following topical 1,25(OH)$_2$D$_3$ may have been due to the apoptosis of the cells, and/or their migration into the SDLN. In preliminary studies, we have observed significant increases (by a mean of 27±15%, mean±SEM, n=4 experiments) in the numbers of skin-derived DC (CD11c+MHCII+DEC-205^{hi}CD8^{lo} cells) [25] in the SDLN 18 h after 1,25(OH)$_2$D$_3$ (125 ng) application suggesting that 1,25(OH)$_2$D$_3$ can induce the migration of DC from the skin into the SDLN. Topical 1,25(OH)$_2$D$_3$ may even promote the migration of skin DC beyond the SDLN, as 1,25(OH)$_2$D$_3$-treated bone marrow-derived DC preferentially migrated into the Peyer's patches after adoptive transfer (either intravenously or intradermally) when administered with diptheria toxin [26].

Effects on Local Contact Hypersensitivity Responses

Reduced DC numbers in the skin have previously been linked to the induction of regulatory T cells and subsequent suppressed 'local' immune responses following the treatment of skin with agents such as UV irradiation [27]. In particular, reductions of skin DC have been associated with suppressed contact hypersensitivity (CHS) responses, when the antigen is applied to the same skin site as UV irradiation [27]. Similarly, topical 1,25(OH)$_2$D$_3$ (400 ng/day) administered once a day for seven days to BALB/c mice significantly suppressed CHS ear-swelling responses when the experimental hapten (DNFB, dinitrofluorobenzene) was applied to the same skin site as 1,25(OH)$_2$D$_3$ [22]. Skin exposure to calcipotriol (three times daily for three days (1500 ng/treatment)) before transcutaneous immunization with ovalbumin (OVA) protein also reduced CHS ear-swelling responses in mice [23]. In addition, human volunteers treated topically with the vitamin D analogue calcipotriene twice daily had significantly suppressed CHS responses when the hapten (DNCB, di-nitrochlorobenzene) was applied to the calcipotriene-treated site [28]. In contrast to these observations, calcipotriol (5 μg) administered on four consecutive days before or after the sensitisation of BALB/c mice had no effect on subsequent CHS responses when the hapten (OXA, oxazalone) was administered to the same site as calcipotriol [29].

Effects on Systemic Contact Hypersensitivity Responses

Vitamin D has less potent effects on systemic CHS responses, when the antigen is applied to a skin site distant to the treated site. $1,25(OH)_2D_3$ (125 ng) applied to the dorsal skin of BALB/c mice 4 days before sensitisation on the abdominal skin with a hapten (DNFB), had no effects on subsequent CHS responses [unpublished data; Gorman S, Judge MA, Hart PH]. In a recent study para-local or systemic Mantoux reactions were suppressed by topical administration of $1,25(OH)_2D_3$ to the skin of human volunteers [30]. In BALB/c mice, if applied after UV irradiation, topical $1,25(OH)_2D_3$ had an additive effect with UV irradiation to suppress the ear swelling responses to a greater degree than UV alone (unpublished data; Gorman S, Judge MA, Hart PH). However, this effect was not observed in Skh:hr1 hairless mice (albino), where $1,25(OH)_2D_3$ reversed the immunosuppressive effects of UV irradiation on CHS responses [31]. In humans, $1,25(OH)_2D_3$ application immediately following UV irradiation did not reverse the immunosuppressive effects of UV irradation on Mantoux reactions [30].

A fundamental disparity in the mouse strains used may explain the differences in our findings and those previously published [31]. Like Skh:hr1 mice, vitamin D receptor (VDR) knockout mice are also hairless, perhaps indicating that expression of the VDR may be dysregulated in the skin of Skh:hr1 mice. Further, the ability of $1,25(OH)_2D_3$ to reverse UVB-induced immunosuppression in Skh:hr1 mice may occur through the non-genomic "rapid-response" pathway and not through one dependent on the genomic VDR [31]. The presence of the VDR in the skin of BALB/c mice and humans, where calcipotriol also suppresses CHS responses [28,31], may thus enable some of the suppressive actions of topical $1,25(OH)_2D_3$.

In contrast and more in line with a homeostatic role for vitamin D, topical $1,25(OH)_2D_3$ after UV irradiation consistently reversed the inflammatory effects of UVB irradiation on lymph node hypertrophy, where the number of SDLN cells/mouse was determined 4 days after the initial skin treatment (unpublished data; Gorman S, Judge MA, Hart PH). Therefore, in BALB/c mice, $1,25(OH)_2D_3$ reverses the inflammatory but not the immunomodulatory effects of UV irradiation of skin. The mode by which topical $1,25(OH)_2D_3$ acts to control skin inflammation could occur by reducing mast cell degranulation as 1,24$(OH)_2D_3$ (2 ng) reduced the ear swelling responses induced by intravenous injection of anti-DNP IgE 1 h before ear challenge with DNFB [32].

Topical Vitamin D Modifies T Cell Responses in the Draining Lymph Nodes

Either through direct passage from the skin through the lymphatics, or by interacting with migrating cells (such as DC), other immune cells in the SDLN may be altered by topical 1,25$(OH)_2D_3$. In particular, T cell responses are diminished following topical 1,25$(OH)_2D_3$ treatment. 1,25$(OH)_2D_3$ (1-2 μg) applied to hind footpad dorsal skin five days after foot-pad immunization with hepatitis B surface antigen (HB sAg) modified the ability of draining lymph node (DLN) cells stimulated with anti-CD3 mAb to secrete cytokines (reduced IL-2 and IFNγ, but increased IL-4, IL-5 and IL-10) [33]. Topical 1,25$(OH)_2D_3$ treatment also significantly reduced the ability of OVA-specific CD4+ T cells from OVA-TCR transgenic mice (DO11.10 mice) to proliferate and produce IL-2 when stimulated *ex vivo* [34]. In more recent studies, skin exposure to calcipotriol (3 times daily for 3 days (1500 ng/treatment)) before transcutaneous immunization with OVA protein and CpG adjuvant prevented OVA-specific CD8+ T cell priming [23]. These observations may be explained by the ability of topical 1,25$(OH)_2D_3$ or calcipotriol to modify the suppressive activity or numbers of CD4+CD25+Foxp3+ cells in the SDLN [23,34].

Regulatory Cell Function is Enhanced After Topical Vitamin D

Topical 1,25$(OH)_2D_3$ enhances the suppressive capacity of CD4+CD25+(Foxp3+) cells residing in the SDLN of mice not otherwise exposed to antigen. This effect was maximal four days post treatment with 1,25$(OH)_2D_3$ (125 ng), where CD4+CD25+ cells purified from the SDLN of 1,25$(OH)_2D_3$-treated mice had an augmented ability to suppress the proliferation of co-cultured T cells, and CHS responses when adoptively transferred into naïve mice, compared to cells from vehicle-treated mice [34]. Chronic treatment of mice with calcipotriol and OVA applied to the same site resulted in the expansion of OVA-specific regulatory T cells in the DLN [23].

Chronic topical calcipotriol also increased RANKL (receptor activator of NF-κB ligand) expression by keratinocytes in a VDR-dependent manner [34]. RANKL expression has previously been linked with the expansion of regulatory T cells following UV irradiation [35]. In other studies, topical calcipotriol induced the expression of immunoglobulin-like transcript (ILT)-3 on skin DC in healing psoriatic lesions but ILT3 was dispensable for the capacity of calcipotriol to induce CD4+CD25+Foxp3+ regulatory cells [36].

Topical Vitamin D Enhances Mucosal Antibody Responses

Other reported effects of topical $1,25(OH)_2D_3$ on immune responses include its capacity to modify antibody responses. When $1,25(OH)_2D_3$ was applied to the dorsal skin of the hind footpads of mice five days after immunization with HB sAg (with aluminium hydroxide also applied as an adjuvant), increased serum and mucosal (vaginal) levels of anti-HB sAg antibodies (IgG, IgA) were detected after both the initial and secondary immunizations [33]. In addition, $1,25(OH)_2D_3$ administered as part of an intradermal vaccination with diptheria toxin augmented mucosal but not systemic DT-specific IgA antibody responses. The ability of topical $1,25(OH)_2D_3$ to enhance mucosal antibody responses could occur by promoting the migration of DC to the Peyers patches [26].

Effects of Topical Vitamin D on Other Diseases

Topical vitamin D may affect the pathogenesis of a number of other diseases, highlighting its potential as a therapy for more that just inflammatory skin diseases like psoriasis.

Skin Cancer

Topical $1,25(OH)_2D_3$ and other vitamin D analogues may affect skin cancer progression. Topical $1,25(OH)_2D_3$ reduced the number of skin tumours induced by 12-*O*-tetradecanoylphorbol-13-acetate [37]. In addition, in a small clinical study, topical calcipotriol reduced the number of actinic keratosis, a precancerous lesion of the skin, in nine patients [38]. The mechanism by which topical $1,25(OH)_2D_3$ affects skin cancers could be by preventing damage to DNA in skin cells. Application of $1,25(OH)_2D_3$ prior to UV irradiation of mouse or human skin reduced the number of skin cells with thymidine dimers and the frequency of sunburn cells in irradiated skin [30,34,39]. In other studies, the vitamin D analogue, tacalcitol was used to effectively reduce the size of a benign skin tumour (senile warts, seborrheic keratosis), which occurs in the elderly [40]. Tacalcitol increased the rate of apoptosis in organ cultures derived from senile warts [40], suggesting that the mode of action of tacalcitol on this skin tumour was through apoptosis.

Breast Cancer

Topical $1,25(OH)_2D_3$ may also have effects on the pathogenesis of breast cancers. In a small clinical trial, topical calcipotriol administered daily to patients with locally advanced or cutaneous metastatic breast cancer reduced the diameter of the treated lesions in 3 out of 14 patients who completed 6 weeks of therapy [41]. Similarly, in BALB/c mice, topical $1,25(OH)_2D_3$ inhibited the growth of a breast tumour (EMT-6) in mice topically administered $1,25(OH)_2D_3$ immediately following injection (subcutaneous) with EMT-6 cells [42]. $1,25(OH)_2D_3$ was administered daily for 5 days and significantly reduced tumour volume in both male and female mice.

Asthma

Finally, recent studies in mice indicate that topical $1,25(OH)_2D_3$ may modulate asthma outcomes and T helper-2 (Th2) type immune responses. In a mouse model of asthma, subcutaneous administration of $1,25(OH)_2D_3$ with ovalbumin as an immunotherapy significantly inhibited airway hyperresponsiveness, ovalbumin-specific IgE levels in serum, airway eosinophilia and Th2 cytokine levels [43]. The effects of $1,25(OH)_2D_3$ as a subcutaneous immunotherapy on asthma responses were mediated by IL-10 and TGFβ [43].

CONCLUSION

Topical vitamin D may control the pathogenesis of inflammatory skin disease by affecting the growth of keratinocytes and skin cells and by regulating immune responses mediated by DC, T cells and other immune cells. Topical vitamin D can also have effects on immune cell migration and inflammatory mediator production in inflamed skin. By effects on DC, topical vitamin D can suppress CHS responses, and perhaps also modulate mucosal antibody responses. Furthermore skin-applied vitamin D can reverse the inflammatory and DNA-damaging but not the immunosuppressive effects of UV irradiation of skin. In different experimental models, vitamin D can also enhance the number and suppressive activity of CD4+CD25+ regulatory T cells. Finally, topical vitamin D may also affect the pathogenesis of other conditions including skin cancer, breast cancer and asthma. Further investigations into the mechanisms by which topical vitamin D acts upon immune cells in the skin and SDLN could help us better understand the pathogenesis of inflammatory skin diseases and perhaps identify new treatments in the future.

REFERENCES

[1] Sigmon J. R., Yentzer B. A. & Feldman S. R. (2009) Calcitriol ointment: a review of a topical vitamin D analog for psoriasis, *Journal of Dermatological Treatment 20*, 208-212.

[2] Lebwohl M., Menter A., Weiss J., Clark S. D., Flores J., Powers J., Balin A. K., Kempers S., Glinert R. J., Fleming T., Liu Y., Graeber M. & Pariser D. M. (2007) Calcitriol 3 microg/g ointment in the management of mild to moderate plaque type psoriasis: results from two placebo-controlled, multicenter randomised double-blind, clinical studies, *Journal of Drugs in Dermatology 6*: 428-435.

[3] Lehmann B. (2009) Role of the vitamin D3 pathway in healthy and diseased skin -- facts, contradictions and hypotheses, *Experimental Dermatology 18*, 97-108.

[4] Rizova E. & Corroller M. (2001) Topical calcitriol -- studies on local tolerance and systemic safety, *British Journal of Dermatology 144, Suppl 58,* 3-10.

[5] Langner A., Ashton P., van de Kerkhof P. C. & Verjans H. (1996) A long-term multicentre assessment of the safety and tolerability of calcitriol ointment in the treatment of chronic plaque psoriasis, *Bristish Journal of Dermatology 135,* 385-389.

[6] Naldi L. & Rzany B. (2009) Psoriasis (chronic plaque), *Clinical Evidence (online)*, 1706.

[7] Gerritsen M. J., Rulo H. F., Van Vlijmen-Willems I., Van Erp P. E. & Van de Kerkhof P. C. (1993) Topical treatment of psoriatic plaques with 1,25-dihydroxyvitamin D_3: a cell biological study, *British Journal of Dermatology 128*, 666-673.

[8] Lu I., Gilleaudeau, P., McLand J. A., Heftler, N., Kamber M., Gottlieb S., Krueger J. G. & Gottlieb A. B. (1996) Modulation of epidermal differentiation, tissue inflammation, and T-lymphocyte infiltration in psoriatic plaques by topical calcitriol, *Journal of Cutaneous Pathology 23*, 419-430.

[9] Reichrath J., Muller, S. M., Kerber A., Baum H.-P. & Bahmer F. A. (1997) Biologic effects of topical calcipotriol (MC 903) treatment in psoriatic skin. *Journal of the American Academy of Dermatologists 36*, 19-28.

[10] Gniadecki R. (1996) Stimulation versus inhibition of keratinocyte growth by 1,25-Di-hydroxyvitamin D_3: dependence on cell culture conditions. *Journal of Investigative Dermatology 106*, 510-516.

[11] Korver J. E. M., Vissers W. H. P. M., van Rens D. W. A., Pasch M. C., Van Erp P. E. J., Boezeman J. B. M. & Van De Kerkhof P. C. M. (2007) A double-blind, randomised quantitative comparison of calcitriol ointment and calcipotriol ointment on epidermal cell populations, proliferation and differentiation, *British Journal of Dermatology 156*, 130-137.

[12] Savoia P., Novelli M., De Matteis A., Verrone A. & Bernengo M. G. (1998) Effects of topical calcipotriol on the expression of adhesion molecules in psoriasis. *Journal of Cutaneous Pathology 35*, 89-94.

[13] Fujimura T., Moriwaki S., Takema Y. & Imokawa G. (2000) Epidermal change can alter mechanical properties of hairless mouse skin topically treated with 1alpha-25-dihydroxyvitamin D3, *Journal of Dermatological Science 24*, 105-111.

[14] von Brenken S., Jensen J. M., Fartasch M. & Proksch E. (1997) Topical vitamin D3 derivatives impair the epidermal permeability barrier in normal mouse skin, *Dermatology 194,* 151-156.

[15] Le T. K., De Mon P., Schalkwijk J. & van der Valk P. G. (1997) Effect of a topical corticsteriod, a retinoid and a vitamin D3 derivative on sodium dodecyl sulphate induced skin irritation, *Contact Dermatitis 37,* 19-26.

[16] Peric M., Koglin S., Dombrowski Y., Gross K., Bradac E., Buchau A., Steinmeyer A., Zugel U., Ruzicka T. & Schauber J. (2009) Vitamin D analogs differentially control antimicrobial peptide/"alarmin" expression in psoriasis, *PLOS ONE 4*, e6340.

[17] Lande R., Gregorio J., Facchinetti V., Chatterjee B., Wang Y.-H., Homey B., Cao W., Wang Y.-H., Su B., Nestle F. O., Zal T., Mellman I., Schroder J.-M., Liu Y.-J. & Gilliet M. (2007) Plasmacytoid dendritic cells sense self-DNA coupled with antimicrobial peptide, *Nature 449*, 564-569.

[18] Penna G., Amuchastegui S., Giarratana N., Daniel K. C., Vulcano M., Sozzani S. & Adorini L. (2007) 1,25-Dihydroxyvitamin D3 selectively modulates tolerogenic properties in myeloid but not plasmacytoid dendritic cells. *Journal of Immunology 178,* 145-153.

[19] Sigmundsdottir H., Pan J., Debes G. F, Alt C., Habtezion A., Soler D. & Butcher E. C. (2007) DCs metabolize sunlight-induced vitamin D3 to 'program' T cell attraction to the epidermal chemokine CCL27, *Nature Immunology 8*, 285-293.

[20] Topilski I., Flaishon L., Naveh Y., Harmelin A., Levo Y. & Shachar I. (2004) The anti-inflammatory effects of 1,25-dihydroxyvitamin D3 on Th2 cells *in vivo* are due in part to the control of integrin-mediated T lymphocyte homing, *European Journal of Immunology 34*, 1068-1076.

[21] Li M., Hener P., Zhang Z., Kato S., Metzger D. & Chambon P. (2006) Topical vitamin D3 and low-calcemic analogs induce thymic stromal lymphopoietin in mouse keratinocytes and trigger an atopic dermatitis, *Proceedings of the National Academy of Sciences of the United States of America 103*, 11736-11741.

[22] Guo Z., Okamoto H., & Imamura S. (1992) The effect of $1,25(OH)_2$-vitamin D3 on Langerhans cells and contact hypersensitivity in mice, *Archives of Dermtological Research 284*, 368-370.

[23] Ghoreishi M., Bach P., Obst J., Komba M., Fleet J. C. & Dutz J. P. (2009) Expansion of antigen-specific regulatory T cells with the topical vitamin D analog calcipotriol, *Journal of Immunology 182*, 6071-6078.

[24] Dam T.N., Møller B., Hindkjaer J. & Kragballe K. (1996) The vitamin D_3 analog calcipotriol suppresses the number and antigen-presenting

function of Langerhans cells in normal human skin, *Journal of Investigative Dermatology Symposium Proceedings 1*, 72-77.

[25] Wilson N. S., El-Sukkari D., Belz G. T., Smith C. M., Steptoe R. J., Heath W. R., Shortman K. & Villadangos J. A. (2003) Most lymphoid organ dendritic cell types are phenotypically and functionally immature, *Blood 102*, 2189-2194.

[26] Enioutina E. Y., Visic D. & Daynes R. A. (2000) The induction of systemic and mucosal immune responses to antigen-adjuvant compositions administered into the skin: alterations in the migratory properties of dendritic cells appears to be important for stimulating mucosal immunity, *Vaccine 18*, 2753-2767.

[27] Schwarz T. (2008) 25 years of UV-induced immunosuppression mediated by T cells – from disregarded T suppressor cells to highly respected regulatory T cells, *Photochemistry and Photobiology 84*, 10-18.

[28] Hanneman K. K., Scull H. M., Cooper K. D. & Baron E. D. (2006) Effect of topical vitamin D analogue on *in vivo* contact sensitisation, *Archives of Dermatology 142*, 1332-1334.

[29] Garrigue J. L., Nicolas J. F., Demidem A., Bour H., Viac J., Thivolet J. & Schmitt D. (1993) Contact sensitivity in mice: differential effect of vitamin D3 derivative (calcipotriol) and corticosteroids, *Clinical Immunology and Immunopathology 67,* 137-142.

[30] Damian D. L., Kim J. Y., Dixon K. M., Halliday G. M., Javeri A. & Mason R. S. (2009) Topical calcitriol protects from UV-induced genetic damage but suppresses cutaneous immunity in humans, *Experimental Dermatology Sept 16* [ePub ahead of print].

[31] Dixon K. M., Deo S. S., Norman A. W., Bishop J. E., Halliday G. M., Reeve V. E. & Mason R. S. (2007) *In vivo* relevance for photoprotection by the vitamin D rapid response pathway, *Journal of Steroid Biochemistry and Molecular Biology 103*, 451-456.

[32] Katayama I., Minatohara K., Yokozeki H. & Nishioka K. (1996) Topical vitamin D3 downregulates IgE-mediated murine biphasic cutaneous reactions. *International Archives of Allergy and Immunology 111,* 71-76.

[33] Daynes R. A., Enioutina E. Y., Butler S., Mu H. H., McGee Z. A. & Araneo B. A. (1996) Induction of common mucosal immunity by hormonally immunomodulated peripheral immunization, *Infection and Immunity 64*, 1100-1109.

[34] Gorman S., Kuritzky L. A., Judge M. A., Dixon K. M., McGlade J. P., Mason R. S., Finlay-Jones J. J. & Hart P. H. (2007) Topically applied

1,25-dihydroxyvitamin D3 enhances the suppressive activity of CD4+CD25+ cells in the draining lymph nodes, *Journal of Immunology 179*, 6273-6283.

[35] Loser K., Mehling A., Loeser S., Apelt J., Kuhn A., Grabbe S., Schwarz T., Penninger J. M. & Beissert S. (2006) Epidermal RANKL controls regulatory T-cell numbers via activation of dendritic cells, *Nature Medicine 12*, 1372-1379.

[36] Penna G., Roncari A., Amuchastegui S., Daniel K. C., Berti E., Colonna M. & Adorini L. (2005) Expression of the inhibitory receptor ILT3 on dendritic cells is dispensable for induction of CD4+Foxp3+ regulatory T cells by 1,25-dihydroxyvitmain D3, *Blood 106,* 3490-3497.

[37] Chida K., Hashiba H., Fukushima M., Suda T. & Kuroki T. (1985) Inhibition of tumor promotion in mouse skin by 1alpha,25-dihydroxyvitamin D3, *Cancer Research 45,* 5426-5430.

[38] Seckin D., Cerman A. A., Yildiz A. & Ergun T. (2009) Can topical calcipotriol be a treatment alternative in actinic keratoses? A preliminary report. *Journal of Drugs in Dermatology 8,* 451-454.

[39] Dixon K. M., Deo S. S., Wong G., Slater M., Norman A. W., Bishop J. E., Posner G. H., Ishizuka S., Halliday G. M., Reeve V. E. & Mason R. S. (2005) Skin cancer prevention: a possible role of 1,25dihydroxyvitamin D3 and its analogs, *Journal of Steroid Biochemistry and Molecular Biology 97,* 137-143.

[40] Mitsuhashi Y., Kawaguchi M., Hozumi Y. & Kondo S. (2005) Topical vitamin D3 is effective in treating senile warts possibly by inducing apoptosis, *Journal of Dermatology 32,* 420-423.

[41] Bower M., Colston K. W., Stein R. C., Hedley A., Gazet J. C., Ford H. T. & Combes R. C. (1991) Topical calcipotriol treatment in advanced breast cancer, *Lancet 337,* 701-702.

[42] Chen G., Baechle A., Nevins T. D., Oh S., Harmon C. & Stacey D. W. (1998) Protection against cyclophosphamide-induced alopecia and inhibition of mammory tumor growth by topical 1,25-dihydrocyvitamin D3 in mice, *International Journal of Cancer 75*, 303-309.

[43] Taher Y. A., van Esch B. C., Hofman G. A., Henricks P. A. & van Oosterhout A. J. (2008) 1alpha,25-dihydroxyvitamin D3 potentiates the beneficial effects of allergen immunotherapy in a mouse model of allergic asthma: role of IL-10 and TGF-beta, *Journal of Immunology 180,* 5211-5221.

In: Vitamin D: Biochemistry, Nutrition ... ISBN: 978-1-61668-273-6
Editor: W. J. Stackhouse, pp. 183-198

Chapter 8

EFFECT OF VITAMIN D_3, K_1 AND B_6 SUPPLEMENTED OIL AGAINST OXIDATIVE STRESS: A STUDY ON FERTILE WOMEN

***Arianna Vignini*[*a], *Francesca Raffaelli*[a], *Alessandro Alidori*[a], *Luca Montesi*[a], *Francesca Petrini*[b], *Laura Mazzanti*[a] and *Laura Nanetti*[a]**

[a]Marche Polytechnic University Ancona, Italy
[b]Fattoria Petrini, Monte San Vito (AN), Italy

ABSTRACT

Oxidative stress is defined as an imbalance between the oxidant and antioxidant systems of the body. Olive oil is the main fat source in the Mediterranean diet which showed a protective role against ageing and/or oxidative stress and related diseases.

In order to investigate such *in vivo* effect on healthy human circulating cells, modifications of oxidative stress markers and platelet membrane fluidity before and after 3 weeks oral supplementation of 20 mL/day with Petrini Plus® were investigated. Petrini Plus® is an organic olive oil enriched with vitamins D3 (1,25-dihydroxy-cholecalciferol), K1 (phylloquinone) and B6 (pyridoxal 5 -phosphate).

* Corresponding author:Dr. Arianna Vignini, Marche Polytechnic University, Faculty of Medicine, Via Tronto 10, Ancona, Italy, Tel. + 39 071 2206058, Fax + 39 071 2206058, E-mail: vignini2@libero.it

15 healthy female volunteers (aged 25–40 years) were enrolled in the study. During phase 1 (3 weeks, T_1) subjects were provided with 20 ml/day of Petrini organic standard extra virgin olive oil, and during phase 2 (3 weeks, T_2) subjects were asked to introduce into their diet 20 ml/day of Petrini Plus extra virgin olive oil.

Thiobarbituric acid-reactive substances level (TBARS) decreased significantly in T_2 compared to both T_1 and T_0 as well as lipid hydroperoxide levels and conjugates dienes. Platelet membrane fluidity tested with probes TMA-DPH and DPH decreased significantly in T_2 compared to T_0 and T_1.

The results of present study suggest that the use, even though for a short period of time, of both Petrini organic standard extra virgin olive oil and Petrini Plus® oil in the diet of fertile women may have a protective effect against oxidative stress and provoke modifications in membrane fluidity of platelets. Moreover, the effects due to the supplementation of the enriched oil are more pronounced, thus confirming an antioxidant role played by the added vitamins (vitamins D_3, K_1 and B_6) and a preventing role against ageing and/or oxidative stress and theirs related diseases.

Keywords: Petrini olive oil, Petrini Plus olive oil, oxidative stress, platelet membrane, fluidity. Running title: Antioxidant effect of supplemented oil on fertile women

INTRODUCTION

It is well accepted that the "Mediterranean Diet" is associated with a lower rate of coronary heart disease (CHD) [1], as well as a reduction in overall mortality [2, 3].

Oxidative stress is defined as an imbalance between the oxidant and antioxidant systems of the body, in favour of the oxidant ones. Oxidative stress produced by free radicals has been linked to the development of several syndromes such as cardiovascular diseases, cancer, and neurodegenerative diseases. Olive oil, the main source of fat in the Mediterranean diet, is a functional food which has been shown to be effective both against oxidative stress associated diseases and ageing [4]. Besides its richness in monounsaturated fatty acids (MUFA) (i.e. oleic acid), olive oil contains minor components with antioxidant properties, such as vitamin E, which exerts its action against lipids and DNA oxidation [5-7].

Olive oil exhibits numerous biological functions which are beneficial for health. A diet rich in MUFA provides an adequate fluidity to the biological membranes, by scavenging free radicals and afford an adequate protection against peroxidation [8].

These antioxidants are also able to prevent the endothelial dysfunction by decreasing the expression of cell adhesion molecules [9], and increasing nitric oxide (NO) production and inducible NO synthesis [10] by quenching vascular endothelium intracellular free radicals [11]. The phenolic compounds, present in olive oil, also inhibit platelet-induced aggregation [12] and have been reported to enhance the mRNA transcription of the antioxidant enzyme glutathione peroxidase [13].

Petrini Plus® is an organic olive oil enriched with vitamins D_3 (1,25-dihydroxy-cholecalciferol), K_1 (phylloquinone) and B_6 (pyridoxal 5'-phosphate).

Vitamin B_6 is well known in its biochemically active form as pyridoxal 5'-phosphate, an essential cofactor of numerous metabolic enzymes. The vitamin is also implicated in numerous human body functions ranging from modulation of hormone function to its recent discovery as a potent antioxidant [14]. In fact, in recent years vitamin B_6 has become a focus of research describing the compound's critical function in cellular metabolism and stress response. However, recently it became clear that it is also a potent antioxidant that effectively quenches reactive oxygen species (ROS) and is thus of high importance for cellular well-being [15].

Moreover also vitamin D_3, together with vitamin E and A, has been shown to act as an antioxidant [16]. In a recent study some authors, while exploring the antioxidative effects of vitamin D in prostate cells, found that the active form of vitamin D, 1 alpha, 25-dihydroxyvitamin D(3), is able to protect non malignant human prostate epithelial cell lines [17].

Furthermore, the hydroquinone of vitamin K1 may act as a potent antioxidant in lipid peroxidation [18].

Thus, the aim of the present study was to measure the thiobarbituric acid-reactive substances levels (TBARS), conjugated dienes, and hydroperoxide content of platelets from 15 healthy female volunteers before and after 3 weeks of oral supplementation with Petrini Plus®, an organic olive oil enriched with vitamins D_3 (1,25-dihydroxy-cholecalciferol), K_1 (phylloquinone) and B_6 (pyridoxal 5 -phosphate).

Human platelets were chosen because they are dependent upon circulating lipids for their membrane lipid content, as they lack a mechanism of synthesis.

PATIENTS AND METHODS

Patients Selection

This two-period crossover study included 15 healthy female volunteers (aged 25–40 years) whose clinical characteristics are summarized in table 1. This study was performed according to the guidelines laid down in the Declaration of Helsinki as revised in 2001 and all procedures, involving subjects, were approved by the Bioethical committee of Marche Polytechnic University. Written informed consent was obtained from all subjects. None of the subjects had any disease. Eligible subjects were also required to have normal screening laboratory values, including complete blood count, prothrombin time, international normalized ratio, and serum chemistry panel. Volunteers with renal or hepatic disease or a history of malabsorption were excluded. Selected subjects had a body mass index in the range of 22–27 kg/m^2, were non smokers and consumed a Mediterranean diet. None of them had a history of alcohol abuse or were taking any drugs known to interfere with calcium homeostasis, vitamin D metabolism or coagulation and the antioxidant systems.

Table 1. Clinical characteristics of the study group (n=15) before (T_0) and after consumption of olive oil Petrini (T_1) and Petrini Plus (T_2).

Subjects	T_0 (n=15)	T_1 (n=15)	T_2 (n=15)
Age (years)	32.5 ± 7.5	32.5± 7.5	32.5 ± 7.5
Body mass index (kg/m^2)	24.5 ± 2.5	23.9 ± 1.7	23.8 ± 1.8
Fasting plasma glucose (mg/dl)	90 ± 10	88 ± 8	88 ± 10
Fasting plasma cholesterol (mg/dl)	160 ± 20	156 ± 14	153 ± 15
HDL cholesterol (mg/dl)	55.1 ± 5.3	59.4 ± 4.4	64.4 ± 3.9*
Fasting plasma triglycerides (mg/dl)	93.3 ± 30.1	91.4 ± 31.4	90.5 ± 27.5

Results are expressed as Mean ± S.D.
*$p<0.05$ T_2 vs. T_1 and T_0

STUDY DESIGN

This is a pilot study because it has been performed on healthy fertile women in order to assess the supplemented oil effects in absence of pathologies.

The study consisted of two dietary phases. During phase 1 (3 weeks, T_1) subjects were asked to introduce 20 ml/day of Petrini organic standard extra virgin olive oil in their diet, and during phase 2 (3 weeks, T_2) this oil was substituted by 20 ml/day of Petrini Plus extra virgin olive oil, which contains vitamin K_1 (0.70 mg/100 ml), vitamin D_3 (50 μg/100 ml) and vitamin B_6 (6.0 mg/100 ml). T_0 represents the time at recruitment.

The composition of tested oils is shown in Table 2.

Table 2. Composition of the tested oils Petrini organic standard extra virgin olive oil and Petrini Plus extra virgin olive oil, enriched with vitamin K_1 (0.70 mg/100 ml), vitamin D_3 (50 μg/100 ml) and vitamin B_6 (6.0 mg/100 ml).

	Petrini (100 ml)	Petrini Plus (100 ml)	Petrini (10 ml)	Petrini Plus (10 ml)	Petrini (% RDA)	Petrini Plus (% RDA)
ENERGETIC VALUE	837 Kcal	828 Kcal	84 Kcal	83 Kcal	-	-
PROTEINS	0 g	0 g	0 g	0 g	-	-
CARBOHIDRATES	0 g	0 g	0 g	0 g		-
FAT among which:	93.3 g	92.0 g	9.33 g	9.20 g		
SATURATED	13.3 g	13.8 g	1.33 g	1.38 g	-	-
MONOUNSATURATED	66.6 g	69.0 g	6.66 g	6.90 g		
POLYUNSATURATED	13.3 g	9.20 g	1.33 g	0.92 g		
VITAMIN D_3	-	50 mcg	-	5 mcg	-	100 %
VITAMIN K_1	-	0,70 mg	-	0.07 mg	-	100 %
VITAMIN B_6	-	6,0 mg	-	0.60 mg	-	30 %
VITAMIN E (natural)	30 mg	30 mg	3 mg	3 mg	30 %	30 %

RDA: Recommended Daily Allowance

Subjects were asked to consume a standard diet (with the aid of a list that was given to them) during the 6 weeks of the study in order to reduce possible interferences; the restricted foods were: green vegetables (such as spinach, broccoli), meat and fermented foods, like cheese, as they are sources of vitamin K. The prescribed diet was a slightly hypocaloric Mediterranean diet (1500 Kcal/day; 18% proteins, 27% lipids, 55% carbohydrates). Subjects were interviewed every 3 weeks to verify that they were following the diet correctly, and that they did not change their oil intake over time. The principal criterion in designing the diet was to approximate the current recommended dietary allowance for vitamin K by providing 65–70 mg phylloquinone/day.

PLASMA ISOLATION

Overnight fasting venous blood samples were collected without haemostasis, in the resting state, between 8 and 9 AM to overcome diurnal variation and were immediately processed. Anticoagulant heparin and citrate dextrose (ACD: 36 ml citric acid, 5 mmol/l KCl, 90 mmol/l NaCl, 5 mmoL/1 glucose and 10 mmol/l ethylenediamine tetracetate, pH 6.8) added tubes were used.

Plasma was obtained at baseline T_0 and at the end of T_1 and T_2. After 10 min of centrifugation (1300 g) at 4 °C, the middle layer of the plasma was rapidly pipetted off and immediately used for the experiments.

In particular, levels of thiobarbituric acid-reactive substances (TBARS), conjugated dienes, and hydroperoxide levels in subjects' plasma were assayed, whilst membrane fluidity was measured in platelets.

PLASMA LIPID HYDROPEROXIDES LEVELS

The levels of lipid hydroperoxides in plasma (100 μg) were evaluated using the FOX assay as described by Ferretti et al. [19]. Briefly, samples were incubated with FOX reagent, then centrifuged at 4.500 rpm for 20 min. The absorbance of the supernatant was determined at 560 nm and hydroperoxide levels were calculated using the molar coefficient (4.3x104 $M^{-}1cm^{-}1$) [19].

PLASMA LIPID PEROXIDATION MEASUREMENT

The degree of plasma oxidation was determined by measurement of the hydroperoxide level of TBARS [20]. TBARS were determined using the method of Yagi [21]. Results are expressed as nanomoles malondialdehyde per 100 μg protein. Proteins were measured by the method of Bradford [22].

Determination of Plasma Conjugated Dienes

Conjugated dienes were assayed by monitoring the increase in absorbance at 234 nm as described previously [23].

Platelet Isolation

Peripheral venous blood was immediately mixed with Platelets were isolated by differential centrifugation in anti-aggregation buffer (Tris-HCl 10mmol/l NaCl 150 mmol/l, EDTA 1 mmol/l, glucose 5 mmol/l , pH 7.4) according to the method of Rao (24). This method involved a preliminary centrifugation at 200 × g for 10 min to obtain platelet rich plasma (PRP). PRP was then washed three times in antiaggregation buffer and centrifuged as above to remove any residual erythrocytes. A final centrifugation at 2000 × g for 20 min was performed to isolate the platelets, which were immediately used for the experiments.

Membrane Fluidity

Platelet plasma membrane fluidity was studied by determining the fluorescence anisotropy (reciprocal of fluidity) of probes 1-(4-trimethylaminophenyl)-6-phenyl-1,3,5-hexa-triene (TMA-DPH), which is incorporated in the lipid-water interface of the membrane bilayer, and 1-6-phenyl-1,3,5-hexa-triene (DPH), which is a totally hydrophobic fluorescent probe [25]. Membrane incubation with TMA-DPH and DPH was performed as previously described [26]. Briefly, 3 μL of TMA-DPH and DPH (10^{-3} mol/L) were incubated for 5 min and 45 min respectively, at room temperature, with 2 mL of platelets' membrane dissolved in 50 mmol/L Tris–HCl buffer solution, pH 7.4. Fluorescence intensity (100 readings each) of the vertical and horizontal components of the emitted light were measured on a Perkin-Elmer LS-50B spectrofluorometer (Perkin-Elmer, Beaconsfield, UK), equipped with two glass prism polarizers (excitation wavelength 365 nm, emission wavelength 430 nm). Steady state fluorescence anisotropy (r) of TMA-DPH and DPH was calculated using the following equation:

r = (IvG- Ih)/(Iv +2Ih)

where G is the instrumental factor that corrects the r value for an unequal detection of vertically (Iv) and horizontally (Ih) polarized light. Fluorescence anisotropy is a quantitative index of the freedom of rotation of the probe; a decrease in the r value indicates a higher mobility of probes in the site where it is located, i.e.,increased membrane fluidity. Sample temperature was maintained at 37 °C using an external bath circulator (Haake F3).

Statistical Analysis

Statistical analysis was performed using SAS statistical package (Statistical Analysis System Institute, Cary NC). All experiments were carried out in duplicate and were usually repeated three times. Results are expressed as means ± standard deviation (SD). The differences between baseline and end-point values within the pooled groups were evaluated using a nonparametric test. The Wilcoxon-Mann-Whitney test was used to evaluate the subjects before and after olive oil consumption. Differences were considered significant with $p< 0.05$.

Results

All 15 subjects completed the study and maintained their weight and waist circumference. Overall, compliance with the nutritional instructions and restrictions given was good, as none of the subjects reported consumption of the restricted foods: green vegetables (such as spinach, broccoli), meat and fermented foods, like cheese, as they are sources of vitamin K. The clinical characteristics of the study group before and after consumption of Petrini Plus® olive oil are shown in Table 1. There was a non significant decrease in BMI, fasting plasma glucose levels, fasting plasma cholesterol levels and fasting plasma triglycerides levels in T_1 and in T_2 compared to T_0, while there was a significant increase in HDL cholesterol levels in T_2 compared to both T_0 and T_1 ($p < 0.05$).

TBARS levels decreased significantly ($p < 0.05$) in T_2 (23.472 ± 1.129 nmol/ml), compared to both T_1 (32.435 ± 2.463 nmol/ml) and T_0 (40.166 ± 1.793 nmol/ml) (Fig. 1). Lipid hypoperoxide levels decreased significantly (p

< 0.05) in T_2 (3,258 ± 0,037 nmol/mgprot) compared to both T_1 (5,517 ± 0,051 nmol/mgprot) and T_0 (7,702 ± 0,110 nmol/mgprot) (Fig. 2). Dienes conjugates decreased significantly ($p < 0.05$) in T_2 (1,643 ± 0,023 arbitrary absorbance numbers) compared to both T_1 (2,511 ± 0,028 arbitrary absorbance numbers) and T_0 (3,555 ± 0,034 arbitrary absorbance numbers) (Fig. 3).

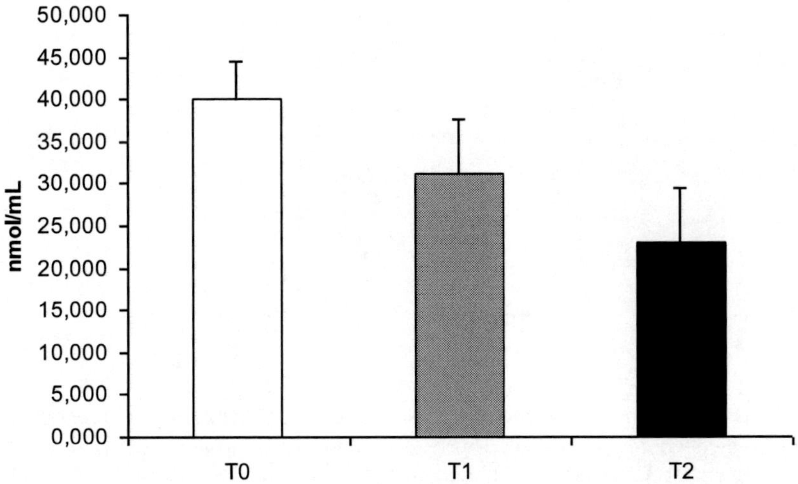

Figure 1. TBARS plasma concentration expressed as nmol/ml in plasma subjects before (T_0), after 3 weeks oral supplementation of 20 mL/day Petrini Oil (T_1) and after 3 weeks oral supplementation of 20 mL/day Petrini Plus Oil® (T_2).

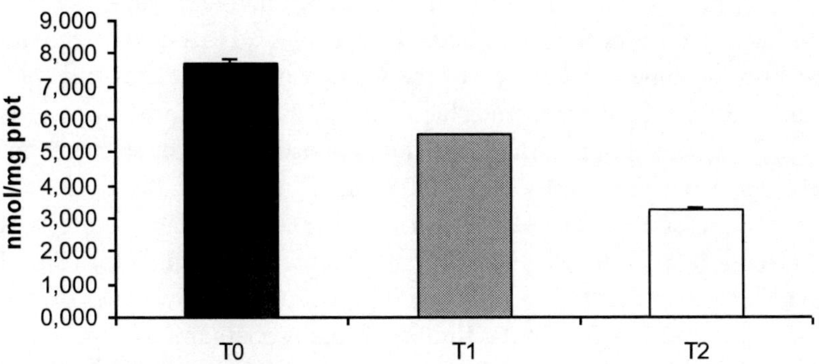

Figure 2. Plasma lipid hydroperoxide expressed as nmol/mgprot in plasma subjects before (T_0), after 3 weeks oral supplementation of 20 mL/day Petrini Oil (T_1) and after 3 weeks oral supplementation of 20 mL/day Petrini Plus Oil® (T_2).

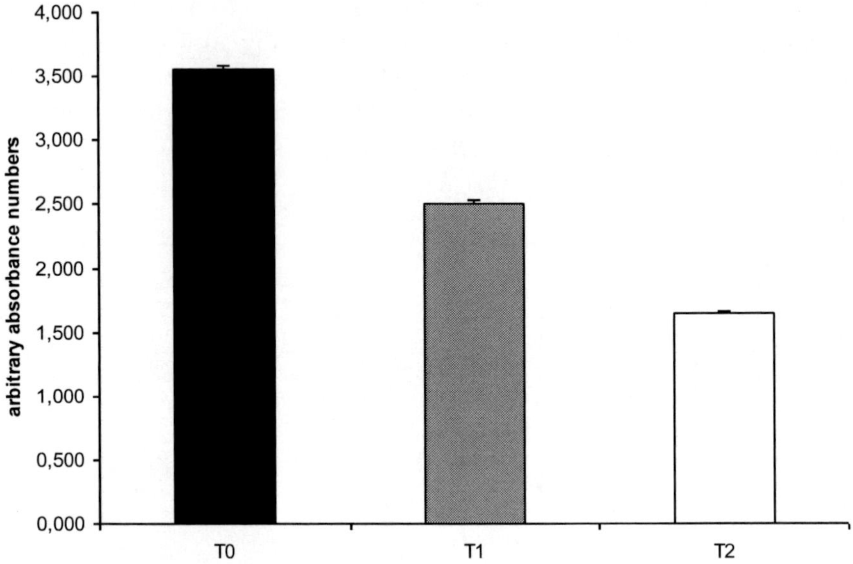

Figure 3. Plasma conjugate dienes expressed as arbitrary absorbance numbers in plasma subjects before (T_0), after 3 weeks oral supplementation of 20 mL/day Petrini Oil (T_1) and after 3 weeks oral supplementation of 20 mL/day Petrini Plus Oil® (T_2).

Membrane fluidity tested with probes TMA-DPH and DPH, and expressed as anisotropy, decreased significantly in T_2 compared to both T_0 and T_1. In particular, TMA-DPH anisotropy values have been shown to decrease significantly ($p < 0.05$) in T_2 (0,140 ± 0,01 arbitrary fluorescence numbers) compared to T_1 (0,167 ± 0,02 arbitrary fluorescence numbers) and T_0 (0,186 ± 0,01 arbitrary fluorescence numbers) (Fig. 4). TMA-DPH provides information on the superficial region of the platelet membrane, having a polar part anchored on the lipid-water interface and on the hydrocarbon tail in the lipid part of the membrane. Similarly, DPH anisotropy values have been shown to decrease significantly ($p < 0.05$) in T_2 (0,194 ± 0,001 arbitrary fluorescence numbers) compared to T_1 (0,197 ± 0,00 arbitrary fluorescence numbers 1) and T_0 (0,199 ± 0,001 arbitrary fluorescence numbers) (Fig. 5). DPH provides data on the deeper, hydrophobic part of the membrane. Because anisotropy is inversely related to the fluidity of the probe's microenvironment, our results indicated a higher fluidity of the external surface of T_2 subjects' platelet membrane.

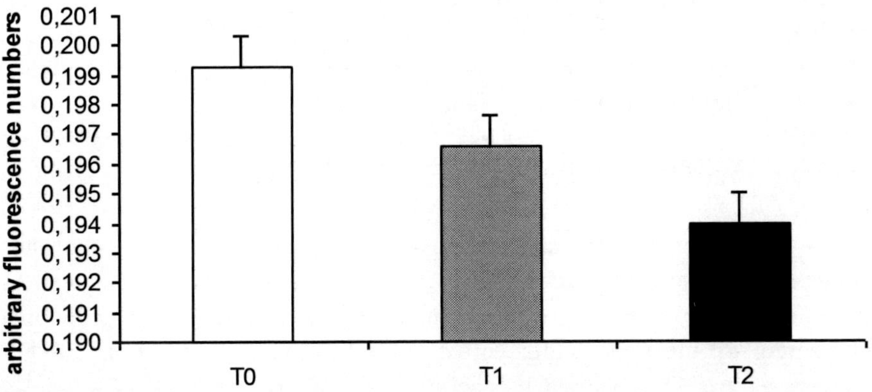

Figure 4. Platelets membrane fluidity tested with probes TMA-DPH and expressed like anisotropy (arbitrary fluorescence numbers) before (T_0), after 3 weeks oral supplementation of 20 mL/day Petrini Oil (T_1) and after 3 weeks oral supplementation of 20 mL/day Petrini Plus Oil® (T_2).

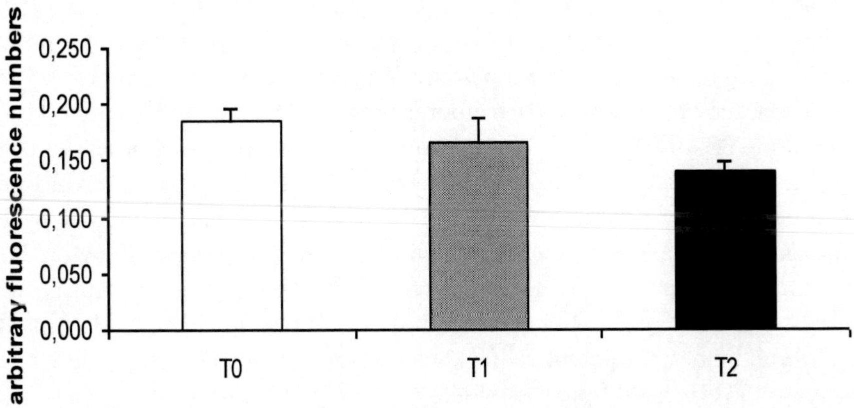

Figure 5. Platelets membrane fluidity tested with probes DPH and expressed like anisotropy (arbitrary fluorescence numbers) before (T_0), after 3 weeks oral supplementation of 20 mL/day Petrini Oil (T_1) and after 3 weeks oral supplementation of 20 mL/day Petrini Plus Oil® (T_2).

DISCUSSION

There is growing evidence that the Mediterranean diet, in which olive oil is the main source of fat, has a beneficial effect on oxidative damage associated diseases such as CHD, cancer, and aging [27, 28].

Phenolic compounds are antioxidant agents present in several foods of the Mediterranean diet among which virgin olive oil. The biological benefits of olive oil consumption in preventing low-density lipoproteins (LDL) oxidation could be linked both to its antioxidant and MUFA content [29].

In the present work these effects were first observed using unsupplemented Petrini organic olive oil, thus confirming previous results [4-7].

Moreover, using Petrini Plus olive oil, an increased HDL cholesterol concentration and plasma antioxidant capacity was demonstrated, as well as a decreased lipid oxidation product content (TBARS), much more pronounced compared to unsupplemented olive oil. A high concentration of HDL cholesterol has been shown to decrease the risk of cardiovascular diseases [30].

In addition, the results of the present study regarding formation of organoperoxides, as determined by the FOX and TBARS assays, might provide a more consistent index of oxidative stress. In fact, oxidative degradation of lipids proceeds by a variety of pathways in which organoperoxides are early products and malondialdehyde is the final product of lipid oxidation [31]. Organoperoxides measured by the FOX assay have also been shown to provide a temporal view of changes in oxidative stress. Regarding TBARS contents, a more pronounced decrease was observed using supplemented olive oil suggesting that the decrease in organoperoxides and lipid degradation products might be due to the antioxidant action of the supplemented vitamins B_6 and D_3 which recent study have been shown to have antioxidant action [14, 15]. In fact recent study indicate that vitamin D_3 may act as a terminator of the lipid peroxidation chain reaction [32], whilst Vitamin K-hydroquinone is a potent radical scavenging species [18, 33] which could decrease the effects of lipid peroxidation.

Moreover, it has been observed that extra-virgin olive oil is able to decrease the prothrombotic environment, modifying platelet adhesion, coagulation and fibrinolysis [34, 35]. In the present paper platelet fluidity, tested with TMA-DPH and DPH probes, was found to be higher after 3 weeks of Petrini and Petrini Plus supplementation. These results might stem from a reduction in overall oxidative stress, due to a decreased membrane lipid peroxidation, which in turn strictly relates to microviscosity, and it is a critical determinant of platelet aggregation and secretion.

In conclusion, data herein reported indicate that the use of both Petrini oil and Petrini Plus oil in the diet of fertile women may have a protective effect against oxidative stress and membrane fluidity in platelets. Moreover, the effects due to the fortified olive oil are more pronounced, thus confirming an antioxidant role played by the added vitamins and a preventing role against ageing and/or oxidative stress and related diseases.

Further studies are in progress in order to clarify the molecular mechanism at the basis of vitamins' action. At present Petrini Plus oil could represent a useful tool against oxidative stress.

ACKNOWLEDGMENTS

The Authors of this research article do not have any conflict of interest at the time of submission.

The present work was supported by Fattoria Petrini, Via San Vito, 12 - 60037 Monte San Vito (AN), Italy, and by ordinary equipment from Marche Polytechnic University to Laura Mazzanti.

REFERENCES

[1] de Lorgeril, M; Salen, P; Martin, JL; Monjaud, I; Delaye, J; Mamelle, N. Mediterranean diet, traditional risk factors, and the rate of cardiovascular complications after myocardial infarction: final report of the Lyon Diet Heart Study. *Circulation,* 1999 99, 779–785

[2] Trichopoulou, A; Costacou, T; Bamia, C; Trichopoulos, D. Adherence to a Mediterranean diet and survival in a Greek population. *Engl J Med*, 2003 348, 2599-2608

[3] Knoops, KT; de Groot, LC; Kromhout, D; Perrin, AE; Moreiras-Varela, O; Menotti, A; van Staveren, W. A Mediterranean diet, lifestyle factors, and 10-year mortality in elderly European men and women: the HALE project. *JAMA,* 2004, 292, 1433-1439

[4] Psaltopoulou, T; Naska, A; Orfanos, P; Trichopoulos, D; Mountokalakis, T; Trichopoulou, A. Olive oil, the Mediterranean diet, and arterial blood pressure: the Greek European prospective Investigation into Cancer and Nutrition (EPIC) study. *Am J Clin Nutr,* 2004, 80, 1012-1018

[5] Fitó, M; de la Torre, R; Covas, MI. Olive oil and oxidative stress. *Mol Nutr Food Res,* 2007, 51, 1215-1224

[6] Masella, R; Vari, R; D´Archivio, M; Di Benedetto, R; Matarrese, P; Malorni, W; Scazzochio, B; Giovannini, C. Extra virgin olive oil

biophenols inhibit cell-mediated oxidation of LDL by increasing the mRNA transcription of glutathione-related enzymes. *J Nutr,* 2004, 134, 785-791

[7] De la Puerta, R; Ruiz Gutierrez, V; Hoult, JR. Inhibition of leukocyte 5-lipooxigenase by phenolics from virgin olive oil. *Biochem Pharmacol,* 1999, 157, 445-449

[8] Alarcón de la Lastra, C; Barranco, MD; Motilva, V; Herrerías, JM. Mediterranean diet and health: biological importance of olive oil. *Curr Pharm Des*, 2001, 7, 933-950

[9] Carluccio, MA; Siculella, L; Ancora, MA; Massaro, M; Scoditti, E; Storelli, C; Visioli, F; Distante, A; De Caterina, R. Olive oil and red wine antioxidant polyphenols inhibit endothelial activation: antiatherogenic properties of the Mediterranean diet phytochemicals. *Arterioscler Thromb Vasc Bio,*. 2003, 23, 622-629

[10] Moreno, JJ. Effect of olive oil minor components on oxidative stress and arachidonic acid mobilization and metabolism by macrophages RAW 264.7. *Free Radic Biol Med*, 2003, 35, 1073-1081

[11] Massaro, M; Basta, G; Lazzerini, G; Carluccio, MA; Bosetti, F; Solaini, G; Visioli, F; Paolichi, A; De Caterina, R. Quenching of intracellular ROS generation as a mechanism for oleateinduced reduction of endothelial activation in early atherogenesis. *Thromb Haemost*, 2002, 88, 335-344

[12] Petroni, A; Blasevich, M; Salami, M; Papini, N; Montedoro, GF; Galli, C. Inhibition of platelet aggregation and eicosanoid production by phenolic components of olive oil. *Thromb Res*, 1995, 78, 151-160

[13] Masella, R; Vari, R; D´Archivio, M; Di Benedetto, R; Matarrese, P; Malorni, W; Scazzochio, B; Giovannini, C. Extra virgin olive oil biophenols inhibit cell-mediated oxidation of LDL by increasing the mRNA transcription of glutathione-related enzymes. *J Nutr,* 2004, 134, 785-791

[14] Fitzpatrick, TB; Amrhein, N; Kappes, B; Macheroux, P; Tews, I; Raschle, T. Two independent routes of de novo vitamin B6 biosynthesis: not that different after all. *Biochem J*, 2007, 407, 1-13

[15] Mooney, S; Leuendorf, JE; Hendrickson, C; Hellmann, H. Vitamin B_6: a long known compound of surprising complexity. *Molecules*, 2009, 14, 329-351

[16] Kolusari, A; Kurdoglu, M; Yildizhan, R; Adali, E; Edirne, T; Cebi, A; Demir, H; Yoruk, IH. Catalase activity, serum trace element and heavy

metal concentrations, and vitamin A, D and E levels in pre-eclampsia. *J Int Med Res*, 2008, 36, 1335-1341

[17] Bao, BY; Ting, HJ; Hsu, JW; Lee, YF. Protective role of 1 alpha, 25-dihydroxyvitamin D3 against oxidative stress in nonmalignant human prostate epithelial cells. *Int J Cancer*, 2008, 122, 2699-2706

[18] Vervoort, LM; Ronden, JE; Thijssen, HH. The potent antioxidant activity of the vitamin K cycle in microsomal lipid peroxidation. *Biochem Pharmacol*, 1997, 54, 871-876

[19] Ferretti, G; Bacchetti, T; Moroni, C; Vignini, A; Nanetti, L; Curatola, G. Effect of homocysteinylation of low density lipoproteins on lipid peroxidation of human endothelial cells. *J Cell Biochem*, 2004, 92, 351–360

[20] Rabini, RA; Fumelli, P; Galassi, R; Dousset, N; Taus, M; Ferretti, G; Mazzanti, L; Curatola, G; Solera, ML; Valdiguié, P. Increased susceptibility to lipid oxidation of low-density lipoproteins and erythrocyte membranes from diabetic patients. *Metabolism*, 1994, 43, 1470–1474

[21] Yagi, K. Lipid peroxides and related radicals in clinical medicine. *Adv Exp Med Biol*, 1994, 366, 1–15

[22] Bradford, M. A rapid and sensitive method for the quantitation of microgram quantities of protein utilizing the principle of protein-dye binding. *Anal Biochem*, 1976, 72, 248–254

[23] Esterbauer, H; Gebicki, J; Puhl, H; Jürgens, G. The role of lipid peroxidation and antioxidants in oxidative modification of LDL. *Free Radic Biol Med*, 1992, 13, 341-390

[24] Rao, GHR. Measurement of ionized calcium in normal human blood platelets. *Anal Biochem*, 1988, 169, 400-404

[25] Duportail, G; Weinreb, A. Photochemical changes of fluorescent probes in membranes and their effect on the observed fluorescence anisotropy values. *Biochim Biophys Acta*, 1983, 736, 171-177

[26] Sheridan, NP; Block, ER. Plasma membrane fluidity measurements in intact endothelial cells: effect of hyperoxia on fluorescence anisotropies of 1-[4-(trimethylamino)phenyl]-6-phenyl hexa-1,3,5-triene. *J Cell Physiol*, 1988, 134, 117-123

[27] Renaud, S; de Lorgeril, M; Delaye, J; Guidollet, J; Jacquard, F; Mamelle, N; Martin, JL; Monjaud, I; Salen, P; Toubol, P. Cretan Mediterranean diet for prevention of coronary heart disease. *Am J Clin Nutr*, 1995, 61, 1360S–1367S

[28] de Lorgeril, M; Salen, P; Martin, JL; Monjaud, I; Boucher, P; Mamelle, N. Mediterranean dietary pattern in a randomized trial: prolonged survival and possible reduced cancer rate. *Arch Intern Med*, 1998, 158, 1181–1187

[29] Marrugat, J; Covas, MI; Fitó, M; Schröder, H; Miró-Casas, E; Gimeno, E; López-Sabater, MC; de la Torre, R; Farré, M. Effects of differing phenolic content in dietary olive oils on lipids and LDL oxidation. A randomized controlled trial. *Eur J Nutr,* 2004, 43, 140–147

[30] Alsheikh-Ali, AA; Lin, JL; Abourjaily, P; Ahearn, D; Kuvin, JT; Karas, RH. Prevalence of low high-density lipoprotein cholesterol in patients with documented coronary heart disease or risk equivalent and controlled low-density lipoprotein cholesterol. *Am J Cardiol,* 2007, 100, 1499-1501

[31] VanderJagt, DJ; Harrison, JM; Ratliff, DM; Hunsaker, LA; VanderJagt, DL. Oxidative stress indices in IDDM subjects with and without long-term diabetic complications. *Clin Biochem*, 2001, 34, 265–270

[32] Lin, AM; Chen, KB; Chao, PL. Antioxidative effect of vitamin D3 on zinc-induced oxidative stress in CNS. *Ann N Y Acad Sci*, 1053, 319-329

[33] Mukai K, Itoh S, Morimoto H. Stopped-flow kinetic study of vitamin E regeneration reaction with biological hydroquinones (reduced forms of ubiquinone, vitamin K, and tocopherolquinone) in solution. J Biol Chem. 267: 22277-81

[34] Turner, R; Etienne, N; Alonso, MG; de Pascual-Teresa, S; Minihane, AM; Weinberg, PD; Rimbach, G. Antioxidant and anti-atherogenic activities of olive oil phenolics. *Int J Vitam Nutr Res*, 75, 61-70

[35] Ruano, J; López-Miranda, J; de la Torre, R; Delgado-Lista, J; Fernández, J; Caballero, J; Covas, MI; Jiménez, Y; Pérez-Martínez, P; Marín, C; Fuentes, F; Pérez-Jiménez, F. Intake of phenol-rich virgin olive oil improves the postprandial prothrombotic profile in hypercholesterolemic patients. *Am J Clin Nutr*, 86, 341-6.

In: Vitamin D: Biochemistry, Nutrition ... ISBN: 978-1-61668-273-6
Editor: W. J. Stackhouse, pp. 199-209

Chapter 9

VITAMIN D AND HYPERPARATHYROIDISM

William Rolston[a], Donald Bodenner[a,b,c] and Brendan C. Stack, Jr.*[a,b]

[a]University of Arkansas for Medical Sciences, Little Rock, AR
[b]UAMS Thyroid Center, Little Rock, AR
[c]Central Arkansas Veterans Affairs Hospital, Little Rock, AR

ABSTRACT

Vitamin D has become an intense topic of interest over the past 10 years. Vitamin D maintains normal blood levels of calcium and phosphorus and also aids in the absorption of calcium. Therefore, low vitamin D levels (25-OH vit D <30ng/mL) result in a reduction in intestinal calcium absorption, transient decreases in serum calcium, skeletal reabsorption, and a compensatory rise in parathyroid hormone (PTH). This is one form of secondary hyperparathyroidism. Recently, research also suggests vitamin D may provide protection from osteoporosis, hypertension (high blood pressure), cancer, and several autoimmune diseases [1, 2]. The recent interest in vitamin D stems, in part, from observations that inadequate levels of vitamin D are widely prevalent in society, with estimates of up to 36% in healthy adults and even higher percentages of elderly and hospitalized patients [3]. The high prevalence has been attributed to poor diet, minimal sunlight exposure, age-related decreases in cutaneous vitamin D synthesis and, possibly, the overuse of sun blocking products during outdoor activity [4, 5]. Hyperparathyroidism, which has a relatively increased prevalence in the

* Corresponding Author: Brendan C. Stack, Jr., MD, 4310 W. Markham St., #543, Little Rock, AR 72205, 501-686-5140, 501-686-8029 (fax), bstack@uams.edu

aging population, can be complicated by co-existing vitamin D deficiency. We will explore the interrelationship between vitamin D deficiency and hyperparathyroidism in this chapter.

INTRODUCTION

Primary hyperparathyroidism will develop in 1 in every 500 women, and 1 in every 2000 men older than 40 years. One hundred thousand new cases are diagnosed annually in the US. As the population ages, the number of patients diagnosed will continue to increase, as the incidence of hyperparathyroidism increases with age [6].

Hyperparathyroidism is defined biochemically as the secretion of excess parathyroid hormone (PTH) by one or more of the parathyroid glands, leading to hypercalcemia in the absence of another cause. A single gland adenoma is by far the most common cause of hyperparathyroidism comprising 75-85% of cases. Double adenoma and 4 gland hyperplasia account for about 10%, and parathyroid carcinoma is rare, occurring less than 1 % of the time [7].

The etiology of primary hyperparathyroidism has yet to be elucidated. There has been an association with ionizing radiation, and survivors of the atomic bomb were 4 times more likely to have primary hyperparathyroidism [28]. There are known associations with multiple endocrine neoplasia syndrome MEN2a, a hereditary disease involving RET oncogene mutations that can cause hyperparathyroidism, medullary thyroid carcinoma and pheochromocytoma.[7]. For the vast majority of primary hyperparathyroidism, it appears to be a spontaneously occurring disease.

The presentation of primary hyperparathyroidism has shifted over the past 40 years. Before the widespread availability of calcium assays, the disease presented much later with more severe symptoms including kidney stones and severe bone disease. Today, between 70-80% of patients are asymptomatic with respect to the classic symptoms of primary hyperparathyroidism such as kidney stones, pancreatitis, and skeletal disease. Non-classic symptoms are more difficult to document and objectify and include fatigue, bone or joint pain, cognitive difficulty, insomnia, and depression, among others. In symptomatic patients, nephrolithiasis remains the most common presenting symptom [7].

The classic diagnosis of primary hyperparathyroidism requires hypercalcemia with an inappropriately elevated PTH and hypercalcuria. Pre-operative planning often involves sestamibi scan with or without SPECT CT and/or ultrasonography. Pre-operative localization has been responsible for both a proliferation in parathyroid surgery and the advent of minimally invasive approaches and improved surgical success rates.

The only cure for primary hyperparathyroidism is surgery. Techniques vary from large incision bilateral neck exploration with identification of all 4 glands to minimally invasive techniques. At our institution, we favor minimally invasive radio-guided parathyroidectomy as described previously by Norman [27]. This involves a preoperative injection of technetium 99-sestamibi and use of intra-operative nuclear diagnosis to aid in identifying the offending gland. Briefly, an excised gland that has 20% or greater of the radioactivity of the background level is defined as an adenoma. It has also been shown that a 50% drop in pre and post excision intra-operative rapid PTH assay levels indicate a cure in the vast majority of patients. These two innovations coupled with improved pre-operative localization have made this surgery very successful, leading to cure 95% of the time in experienced hands [7].

Secondary hyperparathyroidism describes any disorder that results in hypocalcemia and by doing so causes a secondary elevation of PTH levels. Classically this disease is caused by chronic renal failure and the resulting abnormalities in vitamin D, phosphorus and calcium, but vitamin D deficiency is being increasingly identified as a cause of secondary hyperparathyroidism. The mechanism is explained in more detail later, but decreased levels of 25-OH vitamin D lead to decreased levels of activated vitamin D, decreased intestinal absorption of calcium, hypocalcemia and increased PTH levels [5].

As with primary hyperparathyroidism, the presentation of secondary hyperparathyroidism has shifted dramatically due to advances in technology. Classically, patients presented with spontaneous fractures, radiographic evidence of lytic bone lesions, bone pain and extra-skeletal calcifications. Now, patients often present without symptoms due to earlier detection of renal dysfunction and failure [8]. Chronic renal dialysis patients are also screened for this problem regularly.

In recent years there has been an increased interest in vitamin D and its association with hyperparathyroidism. There is a complex interrelation between vitamin D, calcium levels and PTH, and this is the relationship we will explore.

Mechanism

Parathyroid hormone levels are known to be inversely related to extracellular calcium levels. Calcium deficiency up-regulates PTH secretion and cellular proliferation of the parathyroid glands [11, 12]. PTH itself is known to enhance tubular re-absorption of calcium and excretion of phosphorus, and it stimulates the kidneys to produce 1, 25 dihydroxy vitamin D from 25-OH vitamin D via 1- alpha hydroxylase, which increases intestinal re-absorption of calcium [5]. PTH also stimulates osteoclasts to increase release of calcium and phosphorus from bone, causing osteopenia and osteoporosis, increasing the risk for fractures, primarily in the elderly. Calcium, vitamin D and PTH comprise a classic endocrine feedback loop. When slightly above an individuals normal set point, 1, 25 dihydroxy vitamin D and calcium bind to Vitamin D and calcium sensing receptors on the parathyroid cells to inhibit further PTH production. A deficiency of Vitamin D, or hypocalcemia will lead to decreased negative feedback on this mechanism, resulting in decreased absorption of intestinal calcium, triggering an increase of skeletal calcium release, accomplished by further up-regulation of PTH. In chronic renal failure, as renal function declines, there is a loss of available 1-alpha hydroxylase leading to decreased levels of 1,25 dihydroxy vitamin D, decreased intestinal re-absorption of calcium and hypocalcemia. Initially increased PTH levels act to increase phosphate excretion and calcium re-absorption in the kidney, but as GFR levels continue to decline, the ability of PTH to increase phosphate excretion becomes saturated, leading to hyperphosphatemia [9]. Decreased levels of activated vitamin D, hypocalcemia and hyperphospatemia further increase PTH levels.

Over time, chronic PTH stimulation and production leads to hyperplasia of all of the parathyroid glands. Surgically removed parathyroid glands from patients with secondary hyperparathyroidism have been histologically examined and show nodular and diffuse types of hyperplasia [10, 13, 14]. Nodular areas have been shown to be refractory to medical therapy, and over 85% of glands over 500mg show areas of nodularity [15, 16]. Decreased expression of calcium sensing receptors have also been shown in hyperplastic glands, a key component in the negative feedback loop [17, 18, 19]. These absent receptors may explain why PTH levels stay elevated despite normal or high calcium.

Vitamin D Deficiency

Vitamin D deficiency is widely prevalent with up to 36% of healthy patients having decreased levels, and even higher percentages in elderly and hospitalized patients [3]. Three studies showed that a majority of primary hyperparathyroidism patients were either deficient or insufficient preoperatively. Two studies report 61% of patients were Vitamin D deficient or insufficient, and another more recent study showed that up to 75% of elderly patients with primary hyperparathyroidism had coincident vitamin D deficiency [5,20,21]. The importance of vitamin D and its relationship to calcium homeostasis and optimal skeletal growth have long been appreciated. Recently, vitamin D deficiency has also been implicated in contributing to increased risk of breast, prostate, and ovarian cancers. Also hypertension and certain autoimmune diseases seem to be more prevalent in the population with hypovitaminosis D [1, 2].

There are multiple factors contributing to the increasing incidence of vitamin D deficiency. Society has increasingly moved indoors. Sun-blocking skin products have become more popular for protection against skin cancer. The aging population is increasing, and the elderly have a known decreased ability to synthesize vitamin D in the skin. Diets void of vitamin D fortified products are also common [4, 5]. One might expect vitamin D to be implicated in further pathologic processes as they become more prevalent and studied.

VITAMIN D AND HYPERPARATHYROIDISM: ITS CLINICAL IMPLICATIONS

There has been increased interest in the past 10 years on how to apply the knowledge of the complex relationship between vitamin D levels and hyperparathyroidism to clinical practice. As stated earlier, there are a disproportionate number of patients with primary hyperparathyroidism who are vitamin D deficient with these proportions being more extreme in the elderly. We will review recent literature on the subject and describe how it impacts the clinical practice.

It appears low vitamin D may affect the clinical course of the hyperparathyroidism. Beyer et al. showed that patients with vitamin D insufficiency had significantly higher preoperative calcium and PTH levels, as well as bone specific alkaline phosphatase, and intraoperative PTH values. Gland size was also significantly larger in the deficient group. IOPTH values were higher at all time intervals reported in the vitamin D deficient group. The conclusion from this is that vitamin D deficiency is a risk for biochemically more severe hyperparathyroidism which may translate into more severe symptoms and more post operative hypocalcemia [23]. Kandil et al. came to similar conclusions, with lower vitamin D levels causing higher intra-operative PTH levels, higher alkaline phosphatase levels and higher adenoma weight. Interestingly, they also found that patients with hypovitaminosis D were 8 times more likely to have a localizing sestamibi scan [21]. This would likely result in more surgery being performed in this group as opposed to non-localizers. Alternatively, it is less likely that the low vitamin D is creating the false radiographic diagnoses of hyperparathyroidism and resulting in unnecessary surgery.

Eucalcemia with an elevated PTH post operatively from parathyroid surgery can be a common finding, with some authors noting it in as many as 43% of their patients [24]. Our series was 14% [25]. In 2004 Dhillon et al retrospectively reviewed the charts of patients who underwent parathyroidectomy and explored the association with vitamin D levels and PTH pre and postoperatively. Forty-three percent of patients in their series had elevated PTH and eucalcemia postoperatively. These patients also had significantly higher pre and post-operative PTH levels and significantly lower levels of 1,25 dihydroxyvitamin D and a lower ratio of 1,25 dihydroxyvitamin D/25-OH vitamin D. In the patients who eventually normalized their parathormone levels, there was a significant increase in 25-OH vitamin D levels. Both 25-OH-Vitamin D levels and 1,25 dihydroxy vitamin D levels were significantly and inversely related to PTH levels [24].

At our institution, we explored the issue that elevated PTH with normal calcium levels after surgery was also related to vitamin D status. We found that in a population of 55 patients who underwent parathyroidectomy, 13 had elevated PTH postoperatively at 1 week. Four of these patients had elevated calcium levels and persistent parathyroid disease. Eight of the 13 were vitamin D deficient. Replenishment corrected the PTH in those patients who chose to undergo treatment [25]. Beyer et al. examined 86 consecutive patients who underwent parathyroidectomy. Twenty-six patients were empirically treated with calcitriol and calcium carbonate post-operatively. Sixty patients were treated with calcium carbonate alone. The incidence of eucalcemic hyperparathormonemia was significantly lower in the patients who received calcitriol (12%) than the group that did not (37%). Upon multivariate analysis, only vitamin D supplementation and adenoma weight were significant predictors of post operative eucalcemic PTH elevation [26].

Naturally the next question would be whether to replace vitamin D preoperatively or postoperatively. Will vitamin D repletion reduce severity of disease, and reduce the incidence of postoperative eucalcemia with elevation of serum PTH? Postoperative vitamin D replacement is a generally accepted practice, largely due to the above-mentioned findings of Beyer et al and a delay in its recognition [26]. Grubbs et al. sought to determine if preoperative vitamin D replacement was safe and beneficial [21]. Primary hyperparathyroidism patients by definition have elevated serum calcium and it is thought that replenishing vitamin D in these patients could possible lead to severe hypercalcemia. Grubbs et al. did not find this to be the case. Only 5% of patients experienced an increase in serum calcium and this was a mean increase of only 0.65mg/dL total serum calcium. All patients were asymptomatic. Interestingly they did not find a significant difference between the incidence of postoperative eucalcemia with elevated serum PTH between the groups that were vitamin D repleted and deficient. Vitamin D repletion was also not durable at long-term follow up in deficient patients who had been preoperatively replenished. These patients became deficient again once off treatment. Vitamin D replacement with subsequent decrease in serum calcium also seemed to decrease the % IOPTH decrease during surgery [21]. Beyer et al. found the % IOPTH drop to be the same between vitamin D sufficient and insufficient patients during surgery [23]. Grubbs et al. were able to conclude that pre-operative vitamin D replacement is safe though the clinical implications remain unclear.

There appear to be advantages and disadvantages of both vitamin D repletion strategies. Leaving patients vitamin D deficient preoperatively theoretically increases their risks of cancer, fracture, hypertension and some autoimmune diseases. Conversely, vitamin D replenishment has been shown to decrease the size of parathyroid glands, and this could potentially affect preoperative localization studies and surgical results. A smaller gland will be less likely to localize on sestamibi scans and would be more difficult to identify by ultrasound and during surgery. At our institution these studies are often performed before referral, prior to replacement of vitamin D, thus the imaging studies are not affected. It has been suggested that preoperative vitamin D replenishment with subsequent decrease in calcium may cause a smaller percentage decrease in IOPTH, with potential for affecting surgical outcomes by making it difficult to achieve the 50% or greater drop, the criteria most often used as an intra operative marker for biochemical cure [21]. Other studies have not shown this to be the case [23]. The decrease in metabolic activity due to vitamin D replacement could also make radioguided surgery more difficult by decreasing parathyroid gland hormone production, leading to detection of a lower level of radioactivity, possibly leading to excised adenomas not meeting Norman's 20% rule. Grubbs et al did not show a significant difference in the number of patients who showed eucalcemia with elevated serum PTH when replenished preoperatively. Beyer et al. did show a significant difference, with those being replenished post-surgery having a lower incidence of postoperative eucalcemia with elevated PTH.

At our institution, we have been routinely drawing preoperative levels of intact PTH, serum calcium, ionized calcium, magnesium, phosphorus and 25-OH vitamin D. If there has not been imaging prior to these patients presenting to our clinic, we will order technetium 99 sestamibi SPECT CT and routinely combine this with in office ultrasound. If preoperative vitamin D levels are lower than 30 mg/dL, we will replensish preoperatively. Our treatment consists of 50,000 IU of vitamin D2 for 10 weeks with repeat 25-OH vitamin D measurement. If greater than 30 ng/mL patients are maintained on 1000 IU of vitamin D3 daily, if less than 30 ng/mL they repeat the 50,000 IU of vitamin D2 for 10 more weeks and repeat testing. Once repletion has started, we proceed with minimally invasive radioguided parathyroidectomy as described above.

Our study showed that the majority of patients who presented with postoperative eucalcemia and elevated PTH were vitamin D deficient. We were not routinely drawing and replenishing vitamin D preoperatively at the time of the study. We now have made it routine to do so, and though we have not examined and reported this data set, we have not seen hypercalcemia as a result of this practice and have not noticed an appreciable difference in the success of localization studies. There is certainly a need for randomized, prospective studies to determine whether pre or postoperative vitamin D replacement will become the standard of care for patients with hyperparathyroidism. These have not been published to date. At this point, it is up to the discretion of the practitioner to determine whether pre or postoperative vitamin D replacement will best serve patients with hyperparathyroidism. The most important thing is that the patient is replenished and placed on maintainance therapy and vitamin D deficiency does not go untreated altogether.

Conclusion

There is a significant relationship between vitamin D deficiency and hyperparathyroidism with a complex interaction involving parathyroid hormone. It is not yet known if vitamin D deficiency is a result of primary hyperparathyroidism, co-exists with hyperparathyroidism because of similar patient populations which are effected by both of these conditions, or may predispose one to hyperparathyroidism. Vitamin D replacement does seem to be effective at decreasing confusion with elevated PTH and eucalcemia following parathyroid surgery. Prospective studies need to be performed to explore when vitamin D replacement should be performed and what effects this will have on parathyroidectomy.

References

[1] Holick MF. Sunlight and vitamin D for bone health and prevention of autoimmune diseases, cancers, and cardiovascular disease. *Am J Clin Nutr* 2004;80:1678S-1688.

[2] Edlich R, Mason SS, Chase ME, et al. Scientific documentation of the relationship of vitamin D deficiency and the development of cancer. *J Envirn Pathol Toxicol Oncol* 2009;28(2):133-141.

[3] Holick MF. High prevalence of vitamin D inadequacy and implications for health. *Mayo Clin Proc* 2006;81:353-373.

[4] Holick MF. Vitamin D the underappreciated D-lightful hormone that is important for skeletal and cellular health. *Curr Opin Endocrinol Diabetes* 2002;9:87-98.

[5] Weaver S, Doherty DB, Jimenez C, Perrier ND. Peer-reviewed, evidence based analysis of vitamin D and primary hyperparathyroidism. *World J Surg* 2009;33:2292-2302.

[6] Lundren GL. Natural history of untreated primary hyperparathyroidism. *In: Textbook of endocrine surgery*; Clark O, Duh Q-Y, Kebebew E, eds., 1997. Philadelphia: Saunders, pp 303-310.

[7] Fraser WD. Hyperparathyroidism. *The Lancet* 2009;374:145-158.

[8] Summers GW. Surgical management of parathyroid disorders. Otolaryngology Head and Neck Surgery 1998;3:2519-2532.

[9] 9.Slatopolsky E, Robson AM, Elkan I, Bricker NS. Control of phosphate excretion in uremic man. *Journal of Clinical Investigation* 1968;47(8):1865-74.

[10] Llach F, Velasquez FF. Secondary hyperparathyroidism in chronic renal failure: pathogenic and clinical aspects. American Journal of Kidney Diseases 2001;38(5 Suppl 5):S20-33.

[11] Russel J, Lettieri D, Sherwood LM et al. Direct regulation by calcium of cytoplasmic messenger ribonucleic acid coding for pre-pro parathyroid hormone in isolated bovine parathyroid cells. *J Clin invest* 1983;72:1851-1855.

[12] Ihimi Y, Russell J, Sherwood LM. Regulation of calcium and calcium and 1,25(OD) 2D3 of cell proliferation and function of bovine parathyroid cells in culture. *J Bone Miner Res* 1990;5:755-760.

[13] Yano S, Sugimoto T, Tsukamoto T *et al.* Association of decreased calcium-sensing receptor expression with proliferation of parathyroid cells in secondary hyperparathyroidism. *Kidney International* 2000; 58:1980–86.

[14] Tokumoto M, Tsuruya K, Fukuda K *et al.* Parathyroid cell growth in patients with advanced secondary hyperparathyroidism: vitamin D receptor and cyclin-dependent kinase inhibitors, p21 and p27. *Nephrol. Dial. Transplant* 2003;18(Suppl. 3):9–12.

[15] Tominaga Y, Tanaka Y, Sato K, Nagasaka T, Takagi H. Histopathology, pathophysiology, and indications for surgical treatment of renal hyperparathyroidism. *Semin Surg Oncol* 1997;13:78–86.

[16] Fukagawa M, Kitaoka M, Yi H *et al.* Serial evaluation of parathyroid size by ultrasonography is another useful marker for the longterm prognosis of calcitriol pulse therapy in chronic dialysis patients. *Nephron* 1994;68:221–8.

[17] Canadillas S, Canalejo A, Santamaria R, et al. Calcium-sensing receptor expression and parathyroid hormone secretion in hyperplastic parathyroid glands from humans. *Journal of the American Society of Nephrology* 2005;16(7):2190-7.

[18] Gogusev J, Duchambon P, Hory B. et al. Depressed expression of calcium receptor in parathyroid gland tissue of patients with hyperparathyroidism. *Kidney International* 1997;51(1):328-36.

[19] Yano S, Sugimoto T, Tsukamoto T, et al. Association of decreased calcium-sensing receptor expression with proliferation of parathyroid cells in secondary hyperparathyroidism. *Kidney International* 2000;58(5):1980-6.

[20] Grubbs EG, Rafeeq S, Jiminez C, et al. Preoperative vitamin D replacement therapy in primary hyperparathyroidism: Safe and beneficial? *Surgery* 2008;144(6):852-859.

[21] Kandil E, Tufaro AP, Carson KA et al. Correlation of plasma 25 hydroxyvitamin D levels with severity of primary hyperparathyroidism and likelihood of parathyroid adenoma localization on sestamibi scan. *Arch Otolaryngol Head Neck Surg* 2008;134(10)1071-1075.

[22] Brown AJ, Zhong M, Finch J, et al. Rat calcium-sensing receptor is regulated by vitamin D but not by calcium. *Am J Physiol* 1996;270:F454-460.

[23] Beyer TD, Chen EL, Nilubol N, et al. Short-term outcomes of parathyroidectomy in patients with or without 25-hydroxy vitamin D deficiency. *Jour Surg Research* 2007;143:145-150.

[24] Dhillon KS, Cohan P, Darwin C, et al. Elevated Serum parathyroid hormone concentration in eucalcemic patients after parathyroidectomy for primary hyperparathyroidism and its relationship to vitamin D profile. *Metabolism* 2004;53(9):1101-1106.

[25] Redman C, Bodenner D, Stack BC. Role of vitamin D deficiency in continued hyperparathyroidism following parathyroidectomy. *Head and Neck* 2009;31:1164-1167.

[26] Beyer TD, Solorzano CC, Prinz RA, et al. Oral vitamin D supplementation reduces the incidence of eucalcemic PTH elevation after surgery for primary hyperparathyroidism. *Surgery* 2007;141:777-783.

[27] Costello D, Norman J. Minimally invasive radio-guided parathyroidectomy (MIRP). *Surg Clin North Am*. 1999;8:555–64.

[28] Fujiwara S. A review of forty-five years study of Hiroshima and Nagasaki atomic bomb survivors. Hyperparathyroidism. *J Radiat Res* (Tokyo) 1991;32 Suppl:245-8.

In: Vitamin D: Biochemistry, Nutrition ... ISBN: 978-1-61668-273-6
Editor: W. J. Stackhouse, pp. 211-216

Chapter 10

INFLUENCES OF VITAMIN D ON PROSTATE CANCER PREVENTION AND BONE HEALTH

Janet Laura Colli
University of Alabama at Birmingham
Birmingham Veteran's Affairs Medical Center

VITAMIN D- COMMENTARY/ SHORT COMMUNICATION

Prostate cancer is a leading cause of morbidity and mortality among men in North America and northern Europe. [1]· Genetics, androgens, dietary and lifestyle factors have been recognized as contributors to risk of prostate cancer [2]· Epidemiological studies suggest associations between environmental factors and prostate cancer risk.

VITAMIN D AND PROSTATE CANCER PREVENTION

Prostate cancer exhibits striking geographical variation, with lower incidences and mortalities in southern latitudes (including China and India), and highest rates occurring in United States, Canada and Scandinavia (countries located in northern hemispheres) [3]. Globally, prostate cancer has higher incidences in countries located in the northern latitudes, and overall has a greater propensity to occur in black and elderly men. These are the same populations most likely to suffer from vitamin D deficiency. Hence it has been hypothesized that low levels of vitamin D (and/or lack of sunlight exposure) may increase the risk of prostate cancer.

Large variations in international prostate cancer incidence and mortality rates suggest that changeable environmental factors exert a role on the etiology of prostate cancer. There are epidemiologic studies which show an inverse relationship between the level of solar altitude and prostate cancer incidence and mortality [3]· Inadequate exposure to sunlight or solar ultraviolet (UV) radiation has been consistently implicated as a risk factor for prostate cancer incidence and mortality in many studies [4]. Further, ecologic analysis of geographic variation in cancer mortality rates suggests that inadequate doses of solar UV radiation cause premature mortality from fifteen different cancers in the United States [5]· Exposure to UV radiation leads to the synthesis of vitamin D in humans which has led to the thesis that a vitamin D deficiency may increase the risk of many cancers.

There is evidence the daily requirements for vitamin D increases with age and also are higher in black patients [6]· This is due to evidence suggesting that the skin of older individuals and blacks cannot synthesize vitamin D as effectively as the skin of younger people, and the vitamin D which is produced is less readily absorbed in the intestine [6] Furthermore, it is important to note that the decrease in serum levels of active Vitamin D lead to an age-related decrease in calcium absorption, which may be as high as 50% [7]. In an affiliate study, prostate cancer was found to occur more frequently in older men in who had documented vitamin D deficiencies. They were able to identify age related declines in enzymes (hydroxylases) responsible for the synthesis of active vitamin D [8] Further evidence supporting vitamin D as a prostate cancer inhibitor, stems from the study which demonstrated black men to have higher prostate cancer rates compared to white men, while their serum levels of Vitamin D where lower than white men [9]. An additional study reviewing data on Vitamin D and prostate cancer, has shown men in the Orient with diets rich in vitamin D (e.g. derived from fish) have lower incidence of prostate cancer; while those with a high dietary intake of dairy products rich in calcium (which depresses serum levels of vitamin D) are associated with a higher risk of prostate cancer [10]. Prospective, randomized studies have demonstrated that vitamin D suppressed metastatic lesions when administered to patients with advanced prostate cancer [11]·

Sources of vitamin D include exposure to sunshine or ultraviolet (UV) irradiation of the skin, dietary intake, and oral supplements. The synthesis of vitamin D in human skin begins with exposure to sunlight (UV) [12]. Vitamin D, obtained by humans from UV exposure or diet, is hydroxylated in the liver to form 25(OH) D (calcidiol), the primary circulating form of the vitamin. Calcidiol is converted to the active hormone 1, 25(OH) 2D (calcitriol) in the kidney and other tissues, including prostate. Calcitriol has been found to hinder prostate cancer cell proliferation and tumor metastasis [13] suggesting protections against both initiation and progression of cancer. Although the biologic evidence for an anti-cancer role of calcitriol is strong for prostate cancer, epidemiological data from prospective studies showed inconsistent associations of pre-diagnostic circulating levels of calcidiol and calcitriol with prostate cancer incidence [13]· It has been hypothesized that this lack of correlation may be a result of genetic differences among males. A recent study [14] found that men with the FokI **ff** genotype were more susceptible to prostate cancer if 25(OH) D levels were low. Levels of vitamin D sufficient to prevent cancer in one person may be insufficient in someone with a different genotype and this confounding factor affecting variations has not been taken into consideration in vitamin D studies. This research demonstrated that genetic differences cause some males to become more susceptible to prostate cancer in the presence of low vitamin D levels. Laboratory data suggests that the active metabolite of Vitamin D (1,25-dihydroxy) inhibits growth of prostate cancer cell lines by inducing cell cycle arrest [15], and inhibits the development of prostate cancer in rat models [16]·

In summary, many studies have identified mechanisms by which environmental and dietary carcinogens might promote prostate cancer [2]· In addition, investigators have recently characterized several susceptibility loci, somatic mutations, chromosomal rearrangements and genetic alterations (deletions and amplifications) involved in the development and progression of prostate cancer [2].The etiology and progression of prostate cancer is most likely a complex interaction between multiple environmental factors and genetic susceptibility. Since it is difficult to alter ones genetic makeup, prostate cancer prevention and treatment largely depends on our ability to alter environmental and lifestyle factors which lead to molecular changes that cause prostate cancer. Large-scale prevention trials are needed to provide final evidence before making dietary or nutritional recommendations. Future studies, evaluating Vitamin D in prostate cancer prevention need to be performed before we can consider initiating chemoprevention with vitamin D.

VITAMIN D AND BONE HEALTH IN PROSTATE CANCER

The function of Vitamin D is to enhance the absorption of calcium and phosphate in the intestines to facilitate the mineralization of bone. Vitamin D's action on bone mineralization, and bone readsoption, is indirect through the stimulation of enhanced calcium absorption from the intestinal lumen into the bloodstream. Patients with metastatic or recurrent prostate cancer are frequently placed on androgen deprivation therapy (ADT) for treatment. Evidence that early androgen-deprivation therapy improves survival has led to increased use of androgen deprivation hormone agonists in men with distant metastases and locally advanced nonmetastatic prostate cancer [17]·

Osteoporosis is an important complication of androgen-deprivation therapy. Deprivation of androgens has been shown to lead to bone loss in men with prostate cancer by decreasing total bone mineral density. A rapid loss of bone-mineral density occurs within the first 6 to 12 months of androgen-deprivation therapy [18]· Dietary vitamin D supplementation of 400-800IU/d causes a cycle similar to naturally occurring vitamin D: there is an increase in serum 25 (OH) D, a decrease in serum PTH, and a decrease in bone resorption; therefore, decreasing the effect androgen deprivation has on bone mass density [7]· Therefore, patients on androgen deprivation therapy should be placed on Vitamin D and Calcium supplementation to reduce the risk of bone fractures secondary to osteoporosis/osteopenia caused by androgen deprivation therapy.

REFERENCES

[1] Jemal A, Murray T, Samuels A, et al. Cancer Statistics, 2003. *Cancer J Clin* 2003; 53: pp 5-26.

[2] Nelson WG, DeMarzo AM, Isaacs WB, Mechanisms Of Disease – Prostate Cancer. *NEJM.* July 24, 2004, 349; 4, pp 366-381.

[3] Hanchette CL, Schwartz GG, *Geographic Patterns of Prostate Cancer Mortality. Cancer*. December 15, 1992, Volume 70, No 12, pp 2861-2869.

[4] Colli JL, Grant WB: Solar ultraviolet B radiation compared with prostate cancer incidence and mortality rates in United States. *Urology* 2008, 71:531–535.

[5] Grant WB: An estimate of premature cancer mortality in the U.S. due to inadequate doses of solar ultraviolet-B radiation. *Cancer* 2002, 94:1867–1875.

[6] Russell RM. Vitamin requirements in old age. *Age Nutrition*. 1992; 3:20-23.

[7] Lips P.Vitamin D deficiency and secondary hyperparathyroidism in the elderly: consequences for bone loss and fractures and therapeutic implications. *Endocr Rev*. 2001; 22:477-501.

[8] John EM, Schwartz GG, Ingles SA, et al. Sun exposure, vitamin D receptor gene polymorphisms, and risk of advanced prostate cancer. *Cancer Research*. June 15, 2005; 65(12); pp 5470-9.

[9] Klein E. Opportunities for Prevention of Prostate Cancer: Genetics, Chemoprevention, and Dietary Intervention. *Reviews in Urology*. 2002; 4 (supp 5); pp S18-28.

[10] Peehl DM et al. Pathways mediating the growth-inhibitory actions of vitamin D in prostate cancer. *Journal of Nutrition*, 133: pp 2461S-2469S.

[11] 11.Schwartz GG, Hall MC, Torti FM, et al. Phase I/II study of 19-nor-1 alpha-25-dihyroxyvitamin D2 (paricalcitol) in advanced, androgen-insensitive prostate cancer. *Clin Cancer Research*. Dec 15, 2005; 11 (24 Pt1): pp 8680-5.

[12] Stein M, Wark JD, Scherer SC. Falls relate to vitamin D and parathyroid hormone in an Australian nursing home and hosteU *Am Geriatr Soc*. 1999; 47:1195-1201.

[13] Giovannucci E: The epidemiology of vitamin D and cancer incidence and mortality: a review (United States). *Cancer Causes Control* 2005, 16: 83–95.

[14] Li H, Stampfer MJ, Hollis JB, et al.: A prospective study of plasma vitamin D metabolites, vitamin D receptor polymorphisms, and prostate cancer. *PLoS Med* 2007, 4:e103.

[15] Peehl DM, Skowronski RJ, Stamey TA, Feldman D, et al. Antiproliferative Effects of 1,25-Didydroxyvitamin D3 on Primary Cultures of Human Prostatic Cells. *Cancer Research*. Feb 1, 1994; 54; pp 805-810.

[16] Carlberg C, Bendik I, Hunziker W, et al. Two Nuclear Signaling Pathways for Vitamin D. *Nature*. Feb 18, 1993; Vol 361, pp 657-660.

[17] The Medical Research Council Prostate Cancer Working Party Investment Group. Immediate versus Deferred Treatment for Advanced

Prostatic Cancer: Initial Results of the Medical Research Council Trial, *British Journal of Urology;* 1997; 79, 235-46.

[18] Shahinian V, Kuo Y, Freeman J, Goodwin J, Risk of Fracture after Androgen Deprivation for Prostate Cancer; *NEJM* Volume 352: 154-164, January 13, 2005.

INDEX

A

B

C

D

E

F

G

H

I

J

K

L

M

P

T

U

V

W

X

Y

Z